100 Herbs of Power

World Herbs, Their Ancestry and Uses

By

John E. Smith

B. A. (Hons.) M:URHP Dip.C.H.

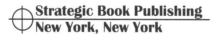
Strategic Book Publishing
New York, New York

Strategic Book Publishing
An imprint of AEG Publishing Group
845 Third Avenue, 6th Floor - 6016
New York, NY 10022
www.StrategicBookPublishing.com

ISBN: 978-1-60693-242-1
SKU: 1-60693-242-X

Printed in the United States of America

Book Design: Roger Hayes

Dedication

To all the great proponents of every healing tradition and to my teachers; past, present and future.

Acknowledgements

My thanks go to my teachers: Michael Tierra L.Ac., O.M.D.
Dr. David Frawley, Hakeem G.M. Chishti,
Maharishi Mahesh Yogi
and Dr. J. Naidu.

My thanks for valuable input to Roy Upton, Andrew Simons, Paul Stamets, Sebastian Pole.

I thank the staff of Earth Force for ongoing support and encouragement.

For patience and willingness to take care of often obscure plants, my wife, Jenny.

For efficiency, patience and technical advice, my thanks to the staff of Strategic Books.

The photograph of Maca from a collection by Oswaldo and Ciro Castillo (permission granted).

Disclaimer

Any health benefits cited in this text are based on centuries of traditional herbal use, and not, unless specified, on modern scientific findings.
The information contained in this book is for educational purposes. It is not intended as an alternative to the advice of a qualified health professional.

Table of Contents

"I came back to life and found myself sitting in the hut of an old Mazatec sorcerer. He told me his name was Porfirio. He said that he was glad to see me and began to teach me certain things about plants that Genaro hadn't taught me. He took me with him to where the plants were made and showed me the mould of plants, especially the marks on the moulds. He said that if I watched for the marks on the plants I could easily tell what they're good for, even if I had never seen those plants before."

The Second Ring of Power – **Carlos Castaneda**

INTRODUCTION

Ancestry

Plants were the earliest land life forms going back (according to fossil evidence) 3.2 billion years.

Those plants were not only our earliest ancestors but also the ancestors of all of the flora and fauna of the present; they carry the genetic memories of everything that has ever existed on planet Earth.

Carbon dating from ancient Babylon (Iraq) records that plants were cultivated as medicines 6,000 years ago.

Written *materia medica* of medicinal herbs go back approximately 5,000 years in India, China and Egypt and at least 2,500 years in Greece and Asia Minor.

Herbs have been used to transform, to diagnose, and to treat spiritual, emotional and physical ills in every tradition from ancient sorcerers of Africa, Mexico and Tibet to the highly regulated medical herbalists of today.

WHAT LIES BEHIND THE HEALING PROCESS?

Do we really know what actually heals?
Or do we simply guess?

We speak of placebo medicine a lot - not only as it relates to natural systems such as homeopathy, etc., but also in terms of pharmaceuticals. We focus our "gospel of what is valid" on "scientific proof" yet we disprove "scientific fact" daily.

We assume that certain herbs are effective either because of their "energetic properties" (e.g. a herb with a descending energy will "ground" a patient, etc.) or because they contain certain nutrients (bio-flavinoids, active ingredients, etc.)

However, it is hard to explain how a rural practitioner with an in-depth knowledge, respect and trust in a small number of herbs can bring about a cure in the most complex and life-threatening disorders.

To paraphrase the naturopath Dr. Christopher, it is better to know a few herbs well than a thousand herbs superficially.

Sorcerers from Mexico speak about "Intent". One of my early trainings introduced many systems of healing. We considered many different approaches to health maintenance including; herbal medicine, aromatherapy, flower remedies, homeopathy, etc. When I asked the tutor what she considered to be the most effective, she replied, "I don't think it really matters what you use. Your intention to make a difference is what really counts."

Perhaps we can give our power to any herb. Perhaps the traditional knowledge behind that herb helps empower it. Or perhaps advanced 'healers' don't need a herb or "totem" and chose whether to use herbs, numbers, names, mantras or mudras.

In the alchemical tradition of herbal medicine; all herbs have numbers that relate to the table of elements. The name of the herb has great significance; not just the common name, such as "**lungwort**" or "**feverfew**", but also its Latin, Sanskrit or Mandarin name (depending on the tradition). For example, "**Solidago**" (**goldenrod**) can be used to develop strength in the past (Solid/Ago). It provides a good foundation for the present and future; Solidago is used as a kidney tonic. (The kidneys are, of course, being behind us).

The herb **Juniper** (Juniperus "communis") can be used to protect against pandemics; the viral or bacterial disorders that affect entire "communities". Traditions as far apart as Tibet and The Navajo Nation, regard Juniper as "The Great Protector.

The above relates to "The Doctrine of Signatures" outlined by Paracelsus in the 16th Century.

I heard of an Ayurvedic practitioner who wrote the name of an herb on a leaf and gave that to his patient as a medicine. Vedic scholars tell us that within the name is the form or that name and form are synonymous.

It is said that Paracelsus ("The Precursor of Chemical Pharmacology") inscribed many of his healing talismans with the names of angels in an obscure script know as "The Alphabet of the Magi".

THE HERBS

The following herbs are some of a vast universal Materia Medica of "totems". We have empowered them with our traditional use, experience and knowledge over the millennia.

CHINESE:

Astragalus, Bupleurum, Cordyceps, Dang Gui (Chinese Angelica), Eleuthero, Fo-Ti, Ginkgo Biloba, Ginseng (Panax), Kudzu, Licorice, Rehmania, Reishi Ganoderma, Schizandra, Tienchi (Sanqi), Wolfberry (Lycium).

AYURVEDIC:

Amla, Andrographis, Asafoetida, Ashwagandha, Bacopa, Ginger, Gotu Kola, Shatavari, Tulsi, Turmeric.

WESTERN:

Cleavers, Coreolus, Dandelion, Echinacea, Equisetum, Garlic, Gentian, Hawthorn, Golden Seal, Milk Thistle, Nettle, Sage, and Yarrow.

OTHER TRADITIONS:

American Ginseng, Californian Poppy, Cramp Bark, Oregon Grape, Cats Claw, Graviola, Jiaogulan, Kalonji, Kava-Kava, Maca, Nigella, Noni, Oudh, Pau D'Arco, Quebra Pedra, Rose, Suma, and Usnea.

THE HISTORY OF HERBAL MEDICINE

In The East

Evidence found in Iraq shows that herbs were grown for medicinal use as early as 6,000 years B.C.

The dates of the first Chinese materia medica ("The Pen T'sao or Classic of the Agricultural Emperor") are vague but most historians fix the date at 2838 B.C.

The Author, Emperor Shen Nung, personally tested 365 medicinal plants.

The earliest texts of Ayurveda (the ancient Indian "Science of Life") were compiled by the physicians Charak and Susrut between 2,000 and 5,000 years before Christ.

Charak wrote in his major text (Charak Samhita):

"Life is just food transformed into life."

In the 1960's, George Oshawa, the founder of macrobiotics (a system based on Eastern tradition) famously said:

"You are what you eat".

Neither Chinese nor Indian herbal medicine was seriously outlawed by church or state. Thus, an unbroken tradition of knowledge has been maintained to the present day.

Avicenna (Ibn Sina), born in 980 A.D., was responsible for more than 270 works including *"The Canon of Medicine"*. This five-volume treatise on healing became the major textbook of all health practitioners for many centuries. It is still regarded by The Encyclopaedia Britannica as,

"the most famous book in the history of medicine".

Avicenna only used natural plant based medicines in balancing what he described as *"intemperaments"*.

In The West

Twenty-five hundred years ago, Hippocrates (the father of medical literature), stated as part of his oath:
"I will give no deadly medicine to anyone".

As a practitioner Hippocrates used only food and herbs, no minerals (except salt), and no synthetic chemicals. Hippocrates is probably best known for the sayings: -
"Let your food be your medicine and let medicine be your food".
"Sickness is caused by the body's inability to digest its environment".

Hippocrates work was influential until the 16th Century when the physician, alchemist and occultist Paracelsus (Philip von Hohenheim) burned the books of Galen and the Persian Master Avicenna in a public square using sulphur to feed the flames.

Paracelsus laid the foundation for allopathic or chemical medicine, as it is practiced today. He was the first western practitioner known to use mercury, or quicksilver, as a prescribed medicine, giving rise to the saying:
"To kill or cure".

The use of quicksilver (quack salver) resulted in medical practitioners being referred to as "quacks".

Paracelsus felt that certain conditions could be rectified by using certain metals. He felt that metals had corresponding planets and organ systems, e.g., gold = the sun = the heart etc.

Paracelsus travelled widely throughout Europe and The East developing his knowledge of alchemy. He created *"The Doctrine of Signatures"*. This relates to the recognition of a plant's properties from its appearance or botanical name.

Paracelsus' studies led him through Europe, Africa and The East. His learning came not only from his Medical training, but from Romany travellers and the Tartar tribesmen who kidnapped him during one of his Eastern journeys.

"Bombastus" was another name adopted by Paracelsus. He certainly appeared to be a bombastic and outspoken character. He came under constant attack and persecution by others of his profession. One story tells of his eventual murder over a difference of professional opinion.

Paracelsus was responsible for inspiring the development of highly potentized herbal medicines known as "spagyrics"; an alchemical system of medicine thought to capture the "soul" and "spirit" of the herb.

Herbalism was outlawed by early allopathic doctors. This was largely through professional jealousy. However, the church played a large part because it believed that healing could only be accomplished by God or his ministers; only monks were allowed to grow, or use, herbs for healing. Other herbalists were often burned as witches.

The American herbalist, Samuel Thompson, was born in 1769. He was a farmer who experimented successfully with local herbs such as **comfrey** and **lobelia** (both now restricted). He was one of the forerunners of a herbal medicine revival. But like early English herbalists of the 15th and 16th centuries, he was persecuted and imprisoned.

Works of Culpepper, Gerard and Thompson, together with more recent herbalists, Hoxsey, Kloss, Treben, Christopher and Tierra, have maintained a tenuous link with the earlier work of Hippocrates.

HERB SAFETY

There are many "Herbs of Power" which I chose not to include in this book because, they can be used inappropriately in the wrong hands. These include: many "psychotropic" herbs, which may be useful in a Shamanic context. They are extremely dangerous when used "recreationally".

The inappropriate use of some simple herbs not only causes problems for the user but also brings the herb, or herbs, into ill repute.

An example is the herb **Ephedra** (Mormon Tea). In wise use it treats asthma and other bronchial conditions effectively. But its stimulating nature gives it "recreational" usage. It has also given ideas to pharmaceutical companies.

A recent U.S. trial of Ephedra's obesity fighting potential showed "favorable results". This in spite of 20-30% of trial participants showing side effects including anxiety and insomnia.

Ephedra use is restricted in The U.K.

Herbs are generally very safe if used wisely or prescribed by a qualified herbalist. Ten thousand deaths per year occur in the United States from taking pharmaceutical drugs as prescribed. [1]

In the United Kingdom deaths linked to Hospital Acquired Infections in patients weakened by antibiotics reach a staggering 6,480 annually. [2] Iatrogenic (doctor caused) death numbers in the United States are greater than those caused by heart diseases (iatrogenic 783,936, Heart Diseases 699,697). [3]

Deaths caused by foods, herbs and dietary supplements are generally considered to be too low to print. [4]

The last figures I have on record (U.K.1991), show approximately 10,000 deaths from prescribed drugs, none from vitamin supplements and 10 (over a 10 year period) from the humble potato.

Unfortunately, the general public is more influenced by the popular press and by flawed research than they are by traditional knowledge. Popular herbs such as **St. John's Wort**

17

and **Black Cohosh** rise and fall in popularity, availability and acceptance according to the whims of the media.

In the following chapters, I attempt to introduce many of the herbs that have stood the test of time.

Notes on Introduction

1. Michael Largo – "Final Exits".
2. The Guardian 29/2/2008
3. Death By Medicine – Nutrition Institute of America – October 2003
4. Roy Law – 2004

PART ONE

CHINESE HERBS IN HEALTH MAINTENANCE AND DISEASE PREVENTION.

It is useful to mention that the Chinese are not preoccupied by viruses and bacteria. They believe that these factors are only worth considering when resistance is low. The major focus in Chinese and most 'traditional' medicine systems is maintaining a state of homeostasis in which the body is strong enough to fight off external pathogens.

Observe Chinese hospitals and you will not see massive use of chemical antiseptics and strong disinfectants. The main "purifiers" I saw in use were rice wine and vinegar. Nor will you bring to light a range of super bugs immune to even the strongest antibiotics.

The average person in China has a rudimentary knowledge of how and what to eat in order to stay well. This knowledge is passed down from an herbal tradition dating back thousands of years.

In Chinese medicine all foods are related to different health conditions and different organ systems; diet is varied according to location, season, climate and individual constitution.

To the Chinese the word herb, is not restricted to medicinal plants but is an umbrella term, which may include: plants, animals, animal parts and by-products, insects, rocks, minerals and resins; in fact anything having a medicinal use. Most Chinese medicines are traditionally taken as part of a meal or in food form (e.g. teas, soups etc.), It is rare for single herbs to be used. Medicinal herbs are used to comprise formulas taking the entire constitution into account.

MAIN ASPECTS OF
CHINESE MEDICINE PHILOSOPHY

YIN & YANG

"Being and non-being produce each other.
Difficult and easy complete each other.
Long and short contrast each other.
High and low distinguish each other.
Sound and voice harmonise each other.
Front and back follow each other."
Lao Tsu

"Both Yin and Yang are only active in the realm of phenomena and have their common origin in an undivided unity"

Willhelm –
The Secret of the Golden Flower

Yin and Yang are the polarities in nature; in harmony they express the underlying value of Unity.

According to Chinese Philosophy there must be an "energetic balance" between the Yin and the Yang of the body for good health and vitality.

Early Taoists were said to have achieved immortality by creating a total balance of Yin and Yang.

The Yin Yang symbol corresponds to the central zone of the wheel of transformation in Hindu symbolism, and to the centre or way out of the labyrinth in Egyptian and Western symbolism.

In the Chinese concept of creation; light and pure substances rise up to form heaven; the grosser substances produce the earth. The two components or powers were called Yang and Yin.

The Yin-Yang school of ancient China, from 400 B.C, set out to explain the principles of creation and destruction in terms of the five elements: wood, metal, fire, water and earth and their interaction with Yin (a female force), and Yang (a male force).

YIN

Yin originally meant *"the shady side of the mountain"*; it is likened to the hidden foundation of a house; it is the support needed to stand strong and steady. Essential Yin diminishes due to overwork, insufficient rest, excessive sexual activity and general ageing.

YANG

Literally translated "Yang" refers to *the sunny side of the mountain"*. It describes the activity that represents a vital life. It is the dynamic action embodying a healthy person.

QI

The universal energy permeates all matter in the way that sap permeates all aspects of a tree. In Japan it is referred to as "Ki" and in India "Prana".

Qi flows through the "dragon lines" and "ley lines" of Chinese and Western geomancy; and the acupuncture meridians of the body.

Qi can be channelled and directed by the martial arts; Qi Gong, Tai Qi, etc., and through the use of herbs and formulae (Qi tonics).

In Chinese Medicine energy is normally described as Qi.

Qi is an unlimited commodity. It only takes on the aspect of limitation in cases of imbalance where energy becomes deficient or blocked. In states of total balance Qi is not experienced; for we only experience energy when we have a sudden surge or lack of it. When energy flows in an uninterrupted way it is such an intimate part of our flesh, blood and bone that there is no actual distinction: it is what we are.

JING

Jing combines with "Original Qi" to form the constitution at the time of conception.

In Chinese medicine Jing relates to the Kidneys and Adrenals.

SHEN

"Shen is the awareness that shines out of the eyes when we are truly awake".

In Chinese medicine Shen relates to the "Spirit of the Heart".

THE HERBS

ASTRAGALUS (Astragalus membranaceus) Huang Qi, Chinese Milk Vetch.

Astragalus is first mentioned in *Materia Medica* of *The Divine Farmers Classic.* It is ascribed to The Agricultural Emperor Shen Nong (1st Century A.D.). It was later classified as a "superior" or "ruler" herb and "a tonic to supplement deficiencies".

Astragalus continues to be used as a primary 'tonifier' in Chinese herbal medicine. It has become known in The West as a major herb for supporting the immune system.

Research: Astragalus is known to support spleen and lung function. It is often used as a "support herb" for patients undergoing radiotherapy and chemotherapy [1]. It is a primary treatment that is combined with other immune system enhancing herbs (such as **Codonopsis** and **ligustrum lucidum**). Studies show a 100% increase in survival time when astragalus complexes are used by lung cancer patients [2].

An increase in angina patient's cardiac output has been measured [3]. together with DNA protection against radiation [4]., and increased sperm motility [5].

Combinations: Standard formulae include the well known Ginseng and Astragalus formula (*bu zhong yi qi wan,*) and Jade Screen *(yu ping feng wan);* the first is used to increase energy while the latter protects from external cold and wind.

Contra-indications: Astragalus should be used with care in cases of excess heat It should be avoided where there is extreme damp or food stagnation.

Acknowledgements: My gratitude to Roy Upton, Herbalist and Editor of 'The American Herbal Pharmacopoeia.

BUPLEURUM: (bupleurum falcatum, Chai Hu, Hare's Ear)

Bupleurum, a perennial Asian herb, is part of the *Apiaceae* or *Umbelliferae* family. It is related to carrot and parsley. Its leaves are said to resemble dill or fennel and it has an attractive yellow flower. It is the root of Bupleurum that is used in Chinese herbalism.

The Chinese name for Bupleurum is "Chai Hu" or "kindling of the barbarians". It is first mentioned in a 1st century B.C. Chinese text.

Traditional Uses: Flu, common cold, fatigue, liver disorders, pre-menstrual syndrome, pain, as a sedative, anti-oxidant, anti-fungal, anti-viral.

Bupleurum is generally used in combination with other herbs for sluggish liver function – referred to as "stagnant liver qi" in Chinese Medicine. This basically means that the "energy" or "qi" is blocked. This is often due to stress or emotional overload. A typical example of this is the formula *xiao yao wan* or "free and easy wanderer". It is one of the most prescribed formulas in Chinese medicine.

Bupleurum appears to work as an immune stimulant by increasing the number of antibody sites on the cell surface and by assisting in the production of interferon [6].

Active Ingredients: Bupleurum contains certain saponins and polysaccharides that are found to have antibacterial [7], anti-tumour [8], and hepato-protective [9] actions.

Drug Interactions: None known.

Precautions: To counteract the over-detoxifying effects of bupleurum it should always be combined with either white peony or scutellaria.

Acknowledgements:
Phyllis A Balch CNC – Prescriptions for Herbal Healing – Avery 2002
Natural Medicines Comprehensive Database – Fourth Edition – Therapeutic Research Faculty 2002
Ron Teaguarden – Radiant Health – The Ancient Wisdom of Chinese Tonic Herbs Warner Books 1998

CORDYCEPS: (cordyceps sinensis, Tibetan caterpillar fungus)

Cordyceps sinensis has been highly valued in Chinese herbalism since 250 BC. It was used exclusively as an aphrodisiac tonic (*The Classic of the Divine Farmer* – circa 200 AD) in the Emperor's court. This use was tested when human clinical trials showed a 64.15% improvement in libido. Subjects were given one gram of cordyceps daily for forty days.[10]

This herb (or fungi) was first found growing from moth larvae in the high meadows of Northern China and Tibet. Its Chinese name *Dong Chong Xia Chao* (which translates as "Summer grass, Winter worm") refers to the fact that its growth cycle peaks in both summer and winter inferring that it supports yin and yang, blood and qi, fire and water *.

Commercially available cordyceps is now cultivated on a grain biomass making it easy to obtain and more acceptable to vegetarians.

Cordyceps traditionally use is to support both lungs and adrenals. A modern application of this herb exemplified this historical use when a Chinese sports coach confessed to using it with his athletic team. They subsequently broke nine world records in the 1993 Chinese national games.

The active ingredients of cordyceps sinensis are a bit of a mystery. Several polysaccharides have been isolated which appear to harmonize blood sugar [11]. Evidence also indicates usefulness in improving liver function [12].

There are few reports of adverse reactions to cordyceps. It is widely available to the general public as a dietary supplement.

Acknowledgements:
Mycology News Vol.1. Edition 3. Sept. 2004
Hobbs.C. Medicinal Mushrooms. Botanica Press 1986
Smith.J. Herbal Roots 2004 The Newsletter of the URHP

* The interdependent, polarities in Chinese Medicine

DONG QUAI: (Dang Gui, radix angelica sinensis, Chinese Angelica, mountain celery)

Dong Quai or Chinese angelica root remains one of the most popular and relied upon herbs for women. It is valued worldwide for supporting a healthy female cycle and easing monthly discomforts.

In Traditional Chinese Medicine (TCM), Dong Quai is classified as a tonic medicine, often referred to as "female ginseng".

Traditional Uses: To rebuild red blood cells in cases of anaemia.

Dong Quai is also used in the treatment of infertility and degeneration of the reproductive system.

It is included in "beauty tonics" to detoxify skin and treat pigment disorders: such as rosacea and vitiligo.

Active Constituents: B.12, folic acid, nicotinamide, biotin, essential oils and polysaccharides.

Contra-indications: Not to be used in cases of breast cancer.

As Dong Quai aids circulation. It is not generally recommended in cases where patients are taking blood thinning, pharmaceutical drugs (e.g. *warfarin*).

In China, as with most Chinese Herbs, Dong Quai is rarely used in isolation but combined with other herbs that support its function: e.g. **white peony and ligusticum**. Commonly used formulae include: *si wu tang* ("4 treasures"), and *ba zhen wan* ("8 precious herbs").

Acknowledgements:

Radiant Health: The Ancient Wisdom of the Chinese Tonic Herbs Ron Teeguarden. Warner Books. New York 1998
American Herbal Pharmacopoeia 2003.
Monograph Dang Gui Root Qu-bing.M. et al (1991)

Advances in the Pharmacological Studies of Radix Angelica sinensis (Oliv) Diels (Chinese Danggui). Chinese Med J. 104(9): 776-781. Zao, K. et al. 2003

ELEUTHERO: SIBERIAN GINSENG: (**Eleutherococcus senticocus**)

"It will keep your virgin face younger
*And prolong your life for ever and ever"**

This Adaptogenic, energy tonic is used to increase stamina and endurance. It has been thoroughly researched by Russian scientists in human trials involving thousands of people in highly demanding jobs, including Olympic athletes.

The Chinese consider Siberian ginseng one of the best herbs in the treatment of insomnia, impotence and stress disorders. It aids in cases of depression by increasing the availability of seratonin ("the happy hormone"). Siberian ginseng is rich in Vitamin A.

This herb originates in Eastern Siberia, China, Manchuria and Korea. It is not a true ginseng but a wild deciduous shrub with a creeping, woody root. It has been used for 2-4000 years in China where it is given the name *ci wu jia.* It is a general tonic to treat low vitality and lack of endurance.

Siberian Ginseng is a close relative of the Chinese herb **acanthapanax**, or *wu jiapi* (known as "bone ginseng").

Numerous clinical trials by Russian researchers established eleutherococcus as an "adaptogen" showing it to assist humans adapt to stressful situations and excel in both physical and mental pursuits.

Siberian Ginseng became very popular in the 1960's when Russian athletes sought ways to increase stamina.

Siberian Ginseng is rich in the glycoside known as eleutheroside. It is also rich in pectins, resins and Vitamin A. Its energy is gentler than **American ginseng** and is a good tonic and restorative for women after childbirth. It is also a useful herb in normalising blood pressure and supporting those suffering from chronic fatigue syndrome.

The name Siberian Ginseng is something of a misnomer as the herb is not a true ginseng although its benefits as an adaptogen are similar. Eleutherococcus has within its botanical name the word "coccus". This relates to its ability to fight bacterial infections: such as staphylococcus, streptococcus etc.

* The above quote is taken from the Poem **Ode to Wujia** by Ye Zhishen (Qing Dynasty) – it may refer to Eleuthero (ci wu jia) or acanthopanax (wu jia pi) or these may be synonymous.

FO-TI: (polyganum multiflorum, *ho shou wu*)

The Chinese name for this herb, (*He shou wu*), translates as: "he's black hair". It refers to a man who lived in the Tang Dynasty whose infertility was cured by Fo-Ti. Chinese legends tell of how if one takes 50 year old Fo-Ti root for a year hair colour will be preserved. If the root is 150 years old it may cause teeth to grow in elderly people. The 3000-year-old root is considered to support earthly immortality - hardly any wonder it is so popular in China.

Whilst doing clinical practice in Nanjing, I mentioned to my tutor, (a well respected professor), that my main interest was rejuvenation and longevity. On my last day in his clinic, he passed me a formula for long life that was recommended by his teacher.

I expected this formula to contain lots of ginseng, cordyceps and other adaptogens. I was surprised to find that the first, major ingredient was Fo-Ti (there are 14 other ingredients in that formula).

Actions: tonic, rejuvenative, aphrodisiac, tissue rebuilding.

Uses: anaemia, impotence, lower back pain, premature greying of hair.

Cautions: should not be used by those with very weak digestion, (unless accompanied by sufficient herbs of a carminative nature).

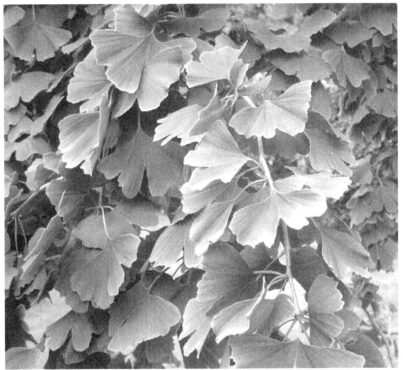

Ginkgo Biloba

GINKGO BILOBA – Maidenhair Tree

One of the world's oldest trees is possibly the oldest living seed plant. Fossil evidence indicates that Ginkgo was well established in the Jurassic period (213 million years ago). Individual ginkgo trees have been known to live for 3000 years. Possibly due to its ancient history and longevity, Chinese and Japanese health practitioners have long associated it with the treatment of age related disorders: e.g. Alzheimer's, etc..

Ginkgo is thought to be an ingredient in the Vedic Elixir "Soma"*, referred to in the ancient Indian texts of Rig Veda.

Over the millennia ginkgo trees developed a powerful immunity to disease and can be found flourishing in polluted inner city areas.

Parts Used: Leaf and Seed

The Leaves act as a vasodilator, stimulating circulation and allowing increased blood flow to the brain to tonify, reduce lethargy and improve memory. A great deal of research exists that shows the effectiveness of ginkgo leaf extracts in the treatment of dementia and hearing disorders, such as tinnitus.

The Seed: Ginkgo seeds are commonly used in Chinese medicine, and are said to be anti-fungal, antibacterial, ant-cancer, and sedative; there are, however, reports of toxicity in high doses.

****Soma**: A ritual drink, used by ancient Vedic cultures similar to the Greek "Ambrosia" and the Persian "Haoma".

Many plants are cited as being ingredients of this elixir including: **Ephedra**, Fly Agaric, Cannabis and Ginkgo Biloba.

Other sources (including Rig Veda), describe Soma as an aspect of divinity or a substance produced naturally in the digestive tracts of enlightened yogis.

GINSENG (Panax trifolium, *ren shen*)

Panax (ren shen) is a deciduous perennial herb. Its fleshy, man shaped root is best used medicinally in the 6th or 7th year of maturity. The most highly esteemed roots, found growing wild in remote parts of Manchuria, are valued at several thousand dollars per mature root.

Ginseng has been known in China for at least 2,000 years; written records of its use go back to 100 C.E.

Panax was reported in "The Classic of the Divine Farmer", as: - an herb to "quiet the essence spirit*, eliminate evil qi**, brighten the eyes, open the heart and prolong life".

Traditionally Panax Ginseng is classified as a spleen and lung tonic. It has a slightly cold energy, (although steam processing the root to produce "red ginseng" lends it a warmer energy). Panax is said to tonify both Yin and Yang. It can be of benefit in all cases of deficiency.

Ginseng is an Adaptogenic herb. That means it use as a self-balanced stimulant / sedative.

Ginseng not only assists in promoting endurance, it also has a relaxing effect on the nervous system enabling the user to function under pressure.

In modern herbal medicine Panax is used as a Qi tonic particularly for the digestive system. It stimulates appetite and corrects prolapse to calm the mind and clear perception.

Scientists (who need to break things down into component parts) have isolated certain saponins in Chinese ginseng, known as ginsenosides. They are thought to have tonic properties; together with polysaccharides known to enhance immune function. It is generally felt that the active ingredients in ginseng are more prevalent in the outer bark and the root-tails of the herb itself and become more concentrated by steam processing.

* Essence Spirit (jingshen) loosely refers to the mind.
**Evil Qi refers to negative environmental factors involved in the cause of disease.

Author's Note:

I feel it is important to add that isolating active ingredients tends to lead to the conversion of harmless herbs to potentially dangerous pharmaceuticals. This gives herbal medicine a bad name. Herbs contain ingredients, which can be described as medicinal. They also contain "buffers" which cushion the effect of the more active ingredients making them safer and more holistic by nature.

Thus Chinese Medicine would rarely use ginseng in isolation. It would be the "Emperor Herb" of a formula including herbs to support, harmonise and direct its function.

JIAOGULAN: (Gynostemma pentaphylum, "Immortality Herb")

Jiaogulan was first recorded in the "Materia Medica for the Salvation of Starvation", in Ming Dynasty China (1368-1644). It was described as "fairy herb", "gospel herb" and "immortality herb" (xiancao). It has wide use in both China and Japan.

A great favourite of mine, it is not only Adaptogenic* but a powerful antioxidant used in the fight against ageing and other "life threatening" disorders.

Jiaogulan (a member of the cucumber family) grows wild in China and other Asian countries where it known as "blue ginseng" because it is similar to ginseng in terms of actions and chemical make-up.

Jiaogulan contains a large quantity of health-giving saponins, (four times as many as ginseng). This helps regulate many bodily systems including blood pressure, reproduction, digestion and the immune system

Chinese research studies show that the use of jiaogulan decreases cholesterol, improves fat metabolism and increases strength and endurance

American scientists have identified Jiaogulan as being one of the ten most effective anti-ageing herbs in the world [13].

A recent Chinese referendum on top healthcare products included three award winning Jiaogulan teas.

Acknowledgements
Blument / Liu, Jiaogulan: China's Immortality Herb. Torchlight Publishing. 1999.

* Adaptogen – A substance that helps the system maintain homeostasis

KUDZU: (pueraria lobata)

On a visit to China in the 1980's research scientist Dr. Lee became interested in a herbal tea formula known as "drunkenness dispelled". This formula centers around the well known herb Kudzu (pueraria).

Kudzu is a creeping plant with starchy roots (the part used as a "food medicine" in China and Japan). It was first recorded in "The Shen Nong", an ancient Chinese herbal text (circa 100 A.D.). It is traditionally used to treat chills, fevers, neck and shoulder tightness and as an alcohol antidote.

Properties: Kudzu is considered to be an anti-spasmodic, diaphoretic, nervine, tonic herb with a vasodilatory action improving blood flow to the brain.

Components: The main active ingredients of Kudzu include the isoflavones: peurarin, daidzin and daidzein.

Daidzin appears to block the enzymes that break down alcohol into its more toxic components, slowing the entry of these toxins into the blood stream and reducing the effects of hangover.

Western history: Kudzu was first introduced into the U.S. as part of a garden design from Japan to commemorate the Centennial celebrations in 1876. It was later used as an ornamental garden plant and used to halt soil erosion. It is now a problem in the Southern States where it has become a noxious weed and has been referred to as "The Vine That Ate the South".

UK PRELIMINARY TRIAL STUDY OF HERBAL FORMULA TO INHIBIT CRAVING FOR ALCOHOLIC BEVERAGES KUDZU COMPLEX

John Smith UK Herbalist
Article Sourced at: http://www.planetherbs.com/

The following preliminary study was conducted in the UK using Planetary Formulas **Kudzu Complex**. It is a formula created by Michael Tierra based on a traditional Chinese formula (TCM) called Ko Ken Tang, with pueraria lobata as the chief herb. The traditional TCM formula is also popularly known as "drunkenness dispeller" for its ability to inhibit the craving for alcohol, reduce drunkenness and the morning after side effects. Thus it is used as an antidote for alcohol. The root of kudzu contains: puerarin, daidzin and daidzein. Daidzin appears to block the enzymes, which break down alcohol into its toxic components, thereby reducing dependency and hangover.

Apart from the Kudzu root and flowers, Kudzu Complex contains other herbs to support, and direct their action, including: **Hovenia** - which also can prevent alcohol toxicity, **Coptis** - an anti-inflammatory, cleansing and liver supporting herb, **Saussurea** - an anti-spasmodic, carminative herb, and **Ginger root** - used for digestive distress, gas and the treatment of nausea.

Many Northern European countries have a problem with over-consumption of alcohol. For the young this is almost considered a "rite of passage." Certainly this is well recognized in countries such as Ireland, Great Britain, Germany and Eastern Block countries; in fact the problem is endemic throughout the European continent. In the UK, sales of Kudzu Complex were steadily increasing and building a steady following amongst customers. The UK distributor of Planetary Formulas, (Earth Force) decided to investigate further the properties of this formula by setting up a trial with eleven people who would take the indicated dose of two tablets of Kudzu Recovery three times daily for a six week period.

The Trial Participants

The trial involved a cross section of people from various backgrounds including: a trainee legal executive, an accountant, a café proprietor and a housewife between the ages of 33 and 63. None would describe themselves as an alcoholic but all found themselves not being able to resist that one last drink "for the road" which often causes aggressiveness and memory loss.

Earth Force's resident herbal practitioner monitored those involved in the trial throughout. At the end of the trial, their general state of health both mental and physical was recorded.

64% claimed to be drinking less and experiencing fewer cravings

55% said they felt and improvement in physical symptoms including: greater energy, less headaches, less symptoms of PMT, less hangovers, etc.

60% said they experienced other improvements including: greater alertness, improved emotional well-being and reduced stress.

Average units per week pre-trial: 36 units
Average units per week post trial: 16 units

40% stated they would like to continue taking the product at their own expense as they were pleased with the results.

During the trial many participants experienced symptoms that could be attributed to the body cleansing itself of toxins. Some felt flu-like symptoms, some felt nauseous and some experienced drowsiness. But in all cases these symptoms subsided.

The two most heavy drinkers found that by the end of the trial that they had either lost the craving completely or were less likely to binge. They were particularly pleased with the results as they had both cut down their consumption of alcohol substantially and felt much better physically and mentally.

The others in this group all felt they could have a drink without it leading to several others as was previously the case. Some found that when under stress, the desire to drink did not materialize as before.

In addition to reducing the craving, along with drinking less alcohol, Kudzu Complex seems to have had a positive effect on concentration, alertness and mood in general.

Conclusion

It is obvious from the above results that Kudzu Complex can be instrumental in supporting a decision to reduce alcohol consumption and thereby improve the quality of life in terms of: improved functioning, greater alertness and reduced stress. As with all dependencies, to be completely successful the individual must be dedicated to changing their drinking habits, not be influenced by peer pressure and be prepared to make a conscious change in lifestyle. Earth Force was genuinely delighted by the results of the Kudzu Complex trial and hope that many more people with drinking problems will choose this natural approach.

Ingredients:

Kudzu flower and root, Hovenia fruit, Coptis root, Poria cocos, Grifola, Atractylodes alba, Codonopsis, Saussurea, Shen-Qu (massa fermentata) Green Citrus peel, Cardamom.

Kudzu Recovery is available in the UK and Europe from many stores that sell herbal supplements or one may contact Earth Force direct info@earthforce.com or Tel. 01873 851953

In the US it is available online from www.planetherbs.com, as well as herb and natural food stores, throughout the country.

LICORICE ROOT: (Glycyrrhiza glabra, G. uralensis)

Uses: A sweet demulcent herb used to treat adrenal deficiency and other glandular problems, good for stomach acidity and all dry lung complaints.

Licorice soothes the gastro-intestinal tract by inhibiting the secretion of gastric acid making it an excellent herb to use in the treatment of ulcers. Licorice is anti-pyretic (fever reducing), dissolves mucous, improves the voice and vision and calms the mind.

In China Licorice is generally used to direct and harmonise a herbal formula and used to detoxify harsher, more bitter herbs; it is known as "the peacemaker" or "the great harmoniser"

Active ingredients: calcium, choline, iron, betaine, magnesium, Quercetin, zinc, and selenium, glycyrrhizic acid, flavinoids, starch, glucose, sucrose, lignums, asparagines.

Licorice is a restorative herb supporting all organ systems (particularly the spleen and lung); it is useful in lubricating mucous membranes, alleviating stress, aiding digestion and assimilation, building blood and energy.

Because liqorice contains substances similar to cortisone it can be useful in treating adrenal deficiencies, and other glandular problems.

Although Licorice is classified as sweet and is 50 times sweeter than sugar, it is still suitable in small quantities for diabetic use.

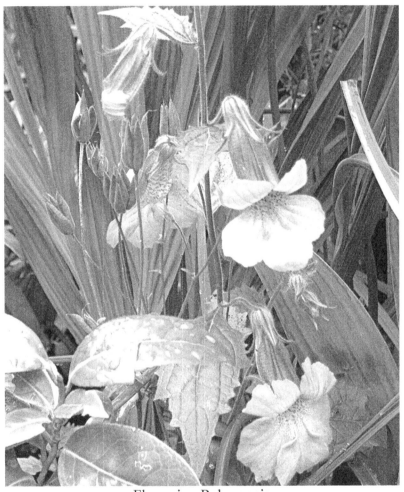

Flowering Rehmannia

REHMANNIA: (Sheng Di Huang, radix rehmannia glutinosa, raw rehmannia, Chinese Foxglove)

The herb Rehmannia can be used either in its raw state (Sheng di huang) or processed in wine (Shu di huang). Sheng di is probably more suitable for yin deficiency as it is cooler in action making it useful in cases of rising fire symptoms, such as thirst, mouth sores, irritability or low-grade fever.

Organ meridians affected: Heart, Liver, Kidney.

Properties: Anti-bacterial, anti-fungal, cardio tonic, diuretic.

Folklore: A Chinese government official claimed Rehmannia was responsible for his being able to father a child at the age of 104.

Actions & indications: Clears heat cools blood – for warm, febrile disorders with red tongue.

Research: 41 out of 50 cases of hepatitis showed significant progress after 10 days of treatment using raw Rehmannia and **Licorice**; results included reduction in size of liver and spleen plus improvement in liver function tests.

All patients in a rheumatology trial using raw rehmannia found marked reduction in joint pain and swelling.

Acknowledgements:
Chinese Herbal Medicine Materia Medica (revised edition) – compiled and translated by Dan Bensky and Andrew Gamble with Ted Kaptchuk. P.69 – Eastland Press. 1993.
The Way of Chinese Herbs – Michael Tierra L.Ac.,O.M.D. p.72 – Pocket Books 1998.

REISHI: "The Mushroom of Immortality", *Ganoderma lucidum,* Ling Zhi.

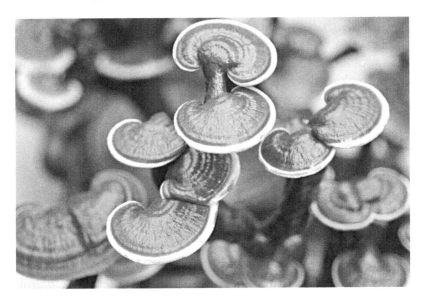

The use of Reishi mushrooms in Chinese Herbal medicine dates back approximately four thousand years.

The first herbal paper on longevity was written on Reishi a mushroom known in China as *"tens of thousand year's fungus".*

Traditionally; reishi is thought to support liver, lung, kidney and spleen function whilst calming the "shen" or spirit (the latter use giving rise to another of its common names: "spiritual vegetable meat").

Reishi mushrooms grow throughout the world particularly on hard woods (oak in The USA, primarily plum in Japan).

The Latin suffix *"lucidum"* (meaning "brilliant") refers to the mushroom's shiny skin giving it a lacquered appearance.

Research on reishi has shown it to have anti-allergic [14]., anti-inflammatory [15], anti-oxidant [16], anti-viral [17]. and anti-tumour [18]. properties; it has also been found useful in the treatment of lung conditions such as asthma and bronchitis [19]..

Many of the findings regarding Reishi are attributed to a class of compounds known as triterpenes, which are reported to have adaptogenic properties.

In both Chinese and Japanese Folk medicine Ling Zhi (g.lucidum) is considered to be in the highest class of tonics.

Contra-indications: Seek advice from a qualified health practitioner if using pharmaceutically based anti-coagulants or immunosuppressants.

Acknowledgements:
Mycology News – Vol.1. Edition 2. Feb. 2000
Hobbs. Christopher – Medicinal Mushrooms. Botanica Press 1986

SCHIZANDRA: (schizandra chinensis, *wu wei zi*, "five flavoured fruit", magnolia vine.)

Wu wei zi literally translates as "five flavoured fruit" as the fruit possesses the five flavours recognised by Chinese medicine (bitter, sweet, salty, sour and pungent); it is generally regarded that each of the five main organ systems of the body responds to a particular flavour – hence schizandra is considered to be a tonic for the whole body.

According to the Emperor Shen Nong (1st Cent. A.D.), schizandra "prolongs the years of life without ageing" and is reported to increase energy, suppress cough, treat fatigue, nourish lungs and kidneys, act as a sexual tonic and calm the spirit [20].. It was considered that schizandra should be taken daily to: "secure and preserve the essential qi and vital warmth of the five internal organs".

In the 13th Century Zhu Dan-Xi, the founder of the "Yin Nourishing School", described this herb as the "protector of youthfulness".

Active ingredients: Schizandra is rich in Vitamin A, C + E, linolenic and linoleic acid and other valuable nutrients.

Research: More than 5000 cases of hepatitis have been treated with schizandra preparations – 75% of cases responded favourably within 20 days [21].

In Russia schizandra is regarded as an "adaptogen" (a substance which reinforces the body's ability to adapt to stress). Various Russian studies have indicated the effectiveness of this herb in speeding recovery time with people exposed to either mental or physical stress [22].

Schizandra was also found to enhance physical performance in racehorses. [23].

Contraindications: schizandra should be avoided in cases of gastric ulcer or epilepsy and either avoided or used with caution during pregnancy.

Acknowledgements: My gratitude to Roy Upton, Herbalist and Editor of 'The American Herbal Pharmacopoeia' (1999)

TIENCHI: (Radix notoginseng, San Qi, "blood ginseng")

Tienchi Ginseng is an anti-inflammatory herb from the South West of China.

Tienchi promotes and regulates circulation and is quite specific for blood clotting, bruises and acute bleeding; so much so that it is the major ingredient in the Chinese formula *"yunnan bai yao"* used in both powder and liquid forms to treat gunshot and stab wounds and general injuries involving trauma.

Tienchi is considered to be the richest of the ginsengs in ginsenosides and is specific for the heart, liver, stomach and colon. As with other ginsengs, Tienchi can vary greatly in quality, is becoming quite rare and is often falsified. Best quality Tienchi is often a rich, black colour, (although indiscriminate dealers, may use boot polish to improve the look of low-grade roots).

WOLFBERRY: (lycium barbaratum, lycium chinesis, "Goji berries" *gou qi zi*)

This sweet red fruit has been prized in China lycium chinensis as a longevity tonic and used by Taoist masters for thousands of years. Li Qing Yuen (1678-1930) referred to wolfberries as being one of the major tonics he used to maintain his life for 252 years.

Lycium fruit is pleasant to taste and can be added to cereals, porridge, pies or wines or merely eaten as a dried fruit snack with nuts and seeds.

It is said that the long-term use of Lycium will brighten the spirit, replenish essence, nourish the liver, enhance fertility and fortify the system against disease

Wolfberry (Lycium fruit) actually contains 124 parts per million of organic germanium demonstrated by Chinese and Japanese studies to be supportive in the treatment of various cancers [24]. perhaps due to its high Vitamin A and Carotene content.

Wolfberry has become extremely popular in the west as a health food. It is sold under the name "Goji".

As an "elixir" (used by the Chinese Empress Dowager) wolfberry is preserved in brandy or rice spirit for 3-6 months and taken in small amounts to replenish "liver blood" and brighten the eyes.

Notes on Part One – Chinese Medicine

1. Wang 1989
2. Morazzoni and Bombardelli 1994.
3. Shi and others 1991
4. Wang and others 1995
5. Hong and others 1992.
6. Estevez – Braun A et al 1994
7. Ahn B Z, Yoon Y D, Lee Y H et al 1998
8. Matsumoto T, Yamada H – Regulation of immune complexes binding of macrophages by peptic polysaccharide from Bupleurum falcatum – 1995.
9. Chui H F, Lin C C, Yen M H et al 1992 - Izumi S, Ohno N, Kawakita T et al 1997
10. Yang.W. et al 1985 Treatment of sexual hypofunction with cordyceps sinensis.
11. Dynamic Influence of Cordyceps sinensis on the Activity of Hepatic Insulinase of Experimental Liver Cirrhosis – Zhang X et al 2004
12. Kodha et al 1985
13. J Nat Prod, 1996: 59: 100-8
14. Chen W American Journal of Chinese Medicine 1996
15. Kiho et al 1986, 1993, 1996, 1999.
16. Lin et al 1993, Stavinho et al 1990
17. Wang et al 1994, Chang & Zhang 1987
18. Kim et al 1994
19. Chen S H et al Studies in the immuno –modulating and anti-tumour activities of
20. Ganoderma lucidum (Reishi) polysaccharides 2004 - Chilton, 1994. Huang 1993
21. Ang 1694, Hsu and others 1986, Bensky and Gamble 1993
22. Chang & But 1983
23. Lupandin and Lapaev 1981, Lupandin 1990, Hancke and others 1996
24. Observation of the Effects of LAK/IL-2 Therapy Combined with Lycium Barbarum Polysaccharides in the Treatment of 75 Cancer Patients, Chunghua Chung Liu Tsu Chih. 1994 Nov.; 16(6): 428-431.

PART TWO

AYURVEDIC HERBALISM IN THE MAINTENANCE OF HEALTH AND THE PREVENTION OF DISEASE

"Avert the danger which has not yet come"
Yogi Patanjali

Ayurveda is probably the oldest health system of the world; it came into being in India's "Golden Age" inspired and influenced by the Vedic scriptures, which are considered by devout Hindus to be the "Blueprints of Creation".

Ayurveda (literally translated as "The Wisdom of Life") is one of the six *Upa* (higher) Vedas and covers various disciplines used to purify the body (including diet, herbal medicine and lifestyle recommendations).

One aspect of Ayurveda, which I feel to be extremely important, is *Rasayana* – the development of elixirs to promote invincibility, increase vitality and prolong life.

AYURVEDA – MYTHOLOGY and HISTORY

AYUR = Life. VEDA (*vid*) = Knowledge, Wisdom.

AYURVEDA is often popularly described as The Fifth Veda

THE VEDAS themselves are known as *apaurasheya* meaning that the texts are not conceived by the human mind but coming from a "divine source".

AYURVEDA is considered to have originated in the mind of BRAHMA the creator who passed it on to PRAJAPATI and from there it was passed to THE ASHWINS (the physicians of the gods) – They passed it on to INDRA (The king of the gods) who gave it to his three Physicians BHARADWAJA, KASHYAPA and DHANVANTARI.

KASHYAPA was reputed to have married the thirteen daughters of PRAJAPATI and fathered all species including animals, humans and demons.

BHARADWAJA was known for his discoveries in aviation. He described three types of flying machine: one that flies from one place to another on earth, one that travels from one planet to another and one that travels from one universe to another;

He also described techniques of invisibility and other powers later cited in Yoga Philosophy.

DHANVANTARI was considered to be a reincarnation of the god Vishnu, often depicted with blue skin (to emphasize his connection to Vishnu) and four arms, carrying a golden leech, a medicinal plant, a conch of wisdom and a pot of rejuvenating nectar.

Dhanvantari wears a *mala* (necklace) of **Tulsi** beads.

The direct disciples of these Mythical Beings were CHARAK and SUSRUT who were responsible for the first major texts of AYURVEDA: The Charak Samhita and The Susrut Samhita.

CHARAK (600 B.C.) described the medical uses of thousands of herbs which modern science is still researching.

SUSRUT (800 B.C) was known largely as a surgeon who specialised in plastic surgery and the removal of cataracts

VEDIC SCIENCE & THE ORIGINS OF AYURVEDA.

The Knowledge covered by Vedic Science is vast and provides the subject matter for many thousands of volumes of texts compiled over a period of at least three thousand years.

The earliest Vedic period of India, responsible for the 1017 hymns of the **Rig Veda,** dates back to an era well before 1000 B.C.; a time when the major Indian civilization was centred around the Indus Valley.

The next period of Indian history (1000 – 600 B.C.) took place in the region between the Himalayas and the mouth of the river Ganges (Bay of Bengal). **Yajur, Sama, Atharva Veda** and **The Upanishads** ("secret doctrine", "milk" or "essence" of the Vedas) were brought to light during that time.

It is generally accepted that Ayurveda was derived from **Atharva Veda:** the Vedic text that deals with rituals and transformation.

From approximately 600 B.C. (the post Vedic period) the six orthodox systems of Indian Philosophy (**Upangas**) together with **Buddhism** and **Jainism** evolved. All of these systems were inspired by the teachings of **The Upanishads,** regarded by Shankara and other great philosophers of that time, as "revealed truth with Absolute authority".

One of these systems known as **Sankhya** was to give form and structure not only to **Ayurveda** but also to **Yoga** Philosophy.

SPICES

Many spice blends used in India have become family secrets and will be added to the cooking of vegetables and lentil dhals, etc. or used as "churnas" (digestive powders taken after food to aid assimilation of nutrients).

TURMERIC: (Curcuma longa)

Turmeric is probably the most underestimated spice from India; it is usually considered more as a colouring agent or dye than as a medicinal herb. However, Turmeric possesses high amounts of curcuminoids, which have "bio-protective" properties both inhibiting the formation of "free radicals" and neutralising those already formed in the body .[1]

A commonly used "churna" in India is the spice blend known as *"Hingashtak"*. Hingashtak is centred around the herb Asafoetida (*Hingu*). This is a root resin rarely found in European stores due to its overpowering smell; earning it the folk name "Devil's dung".

ASAFOETIDA: (Ferula foetida, *"Devil's Dung", "Food of the Gods"*)

Latex, taken from the root of this umbelliferic plant, is dried, ground and usually mixed with rice flour to add to the cooking of beans and pulses. Medicinally this resin is used to aid in the treatment of indigestion, flatulence, intestinal pain, peptic ulcer, parasite infestation and menstrual disorders; it can also be applied externally in the treatment of toothache and acute abdominal pain.

Three other herbs included in Hingashtak are **Ginger**, **Black Pepper** and **Pippali.** These latter herbs also come together to form *Trikatu* (3 Spices), a formula traditionally used in India to clear sinus congestion, improve digestion and break down mucous deposits.

GINGER ROOT: Zingiber officinalis)

Ginger is another great spice herb included in both *Trikatu* and *Hingashtak* and used in traditions throughout the world.

A most versatile herb which benefits stomach, intestines and circulation, Ginger is ideal for nausea, travel sickness, morning sickness (up to 1 gm. daily), colds and flu, pain and disorders involving either mucous or low energy.

Properties: Stimulant, carminative, diaphoretic, analgesic.

Ginger is so highly regarded in both Chinese, and Indian (Ayurvedic) medicine that it is included in more than half of eastern herbal prescriptions; it is used both internally, and externally.

Classified as a "messenger herb" ginger helps to move other herbs through the blood stream to aid absorption and improve effectiveness.

History and Folklore: Ginger was first referred to in the writings of Confucius (500 BC) and used medicinally since that time in both the east and the west.

Chinese mariners chewed Ginger root to avoid scurvy due to its rich Vitamin C content.

Trials: In the early 90's suggested that ginger could significantly decrease the side effects of anaesthetics and other drugs used in surgery.

PIPPALI: (Piper longum) – Indian Long Pepper – *bi bo*

Pippali is a powerful digestive stimulant and a rejuvenative herb useful in the relief of asthma and airborne allergies; it is classified in Ayurvedic medicine as mildly aphrodisiac.

Uses: The fruit of this aromatic pepper is commonly used in the treatment of coughs, colds, tonsillitis, flatulence and diseases of the spleen and liver.

Actions: stimulant, expectorant, carminative, analgesic and aphrodisiac.

Pippali root is also used in decoctions to treat both high blood pressure and insomnia.

Pippali is not dissimilar to the water peppers (smartweed) used by Native American peoples.

BITTERS

All herbal traditions recognise the value of bitter herbs.

Both Chinese and Ayurvedic approaches to health specify the importance of various tastes or flavours (rasas) and how they relate to different conditions and organ systems.

Bitterness is a taste we rarely crave in a Western diet but is nonetheless important.

Herbs such as **Dandelion**, **Golden Seal**, **Coptis** and **Barberry**, etc. fulfil this need and have always been traditional components of "Herbal Bitters" in many cultures.

ANDROGRAPHIS: – The King of Bitters
Other names include: *Kalmegh (Sanskrit) Chuan xin lian (Chinese)*. Chiretta, Andrographis paniculata

Andrographis is a member of the gentiana family. It grows prolifically throughout the east where it is traditionally used to reduce fever and other infections; other areas of use include sore throats, digestive problems, snakebites and malaria (andrographis is a major ingredient in the traditional Ayurvedic malaria powder known as *mahasudarshan churna)*.

It was during the last year of the First World War that andrographis took on a totally new role in helping to overcome the flu virus, which killed 10 million people in India (approx 30 million worldwide).

Modern antibiotic and antiviral medicines not only produce side effects, but also help in the creation of drug resistant "super bugs" whereas potent botanicals such as Andrographis and **golden seal** are generally safe to use when taken as prescribed by a herbalist.

The problem with **golden seal** is that it is now endangered in the wild and (although it is successfully cultivated in the U.S.) is a very expensive herb whereas Andrographis grows abundantly in Northern India, Nepal and certain parts of Africa and (unlike golden seal) can be easily cultivated in the U.K.

In a recent study involving 158 participants suffering from the common cold, Andrographis and a placebo was given daily for four days; by the second day those taking the herb showed significant improvements as compared to those taking the placebo.2.

Andrographis appears to be faster acting than **Echinacea** and is often referred to as "Indian Echinacea" due to its similar actions (including its ability to encourage the production of the cell protein *interferon)*. In Scandinavia Andrographis is more popular than Echinacea and becoming the No.1 flu remedy.

This potent herb can also be likened in action to **Milk Thistle** whose active ingredient *sylmarin* is known to repair liver damage.

All herbal traditions use bitter herbs to reduce fevers and treat toxic heat conditions.

In China the herbs **gentian** and **coptis** are widely used for this purpose, whereas in N.America **golden seal** would be the herb of choice; **cinchona** (known for its active ingredient, *quinine*, is used by the indigenous Amazonian tribes) and European herbalists have traditionally used herbs such as **centaury** and **barberry**. Andrographis is India's contribution to this area of treatment; it is referred to by Ayurvedic doctors as **The King of Bitters** and is used to subdue the *pitta* (fire) *dosha*.

Andrographis can also be compared in action and potency (but without the side effects*) to three commonly used drugs AZT 3., a commonly used AIDS drug, the cancer drug *Tamoxifen* 4., and *loperamine* (*Imodium*) a common drug in the treatment of diarrhoea.

Andrographis has cytotoxic properties giving it potential use in the treatment of cancer. In a 1977 study 12 skin cancer patients given Andrographis all recovered

In a very large study the overall effectiveness in using Andrographis to relieve bacterial dysentery and diarrhoea was found to be 91.3% 5..

I have adopted a particular strategy with regard to strong viruses (especially in the case of those with poor immune function); this involves a short course (5-7 days) of Andrographis (in tablet form – as a tea it is probably the most disgusting herb I have ever tried) followed by a longer course of an immune tonic or protective formula (for example "The Wellness Formula" - Source Naturals, or "Astragalus Jade Screen" - Planetary Formulas). This will generally reduce the symptoms significantly and strengthen resistance.

* The side effects of AZT range from headaches and nausea to reduced red blood cell count. Those of *tamoxifen* include weight gain and hot flushes. Loperimide may cause abdominal distension, pain, nausea and vomiting.

Acknowledgements: Bartameus.P, Andrographis. Health Science. (Newsletter of the Health Science Institute). May 2002.

Pole. Sebastian, Using Ayurvedic Herbs in the Western Clinic (URHP Spring Newsletter) 2003.

Smith.J, Herbal Alternatives to Antibiotic Drugs. Discovering Herbs Newsletter. Autumn. 2002.

MEDHYA RASAYANA: - Elixirs for the Mind

In Ayurvedic medicine there is a sub category known as *medhya rasayana (lit.* elixirs for the mind). The following three herbs, Gotu Kola, Bacopa and Tulsi are certainly featured on that list.

GOTU KOLA: (Hydrocotyl asiatica, Centella asiatica, *Mandukaparni*, Indian pennywort)

Family: Umbelliferae

Gotu Kola is described in India as 'The Meditation Herb' and is said to balance the hemispheres of the brain; it is used to help eliminate excess fluids, decrease fatigue, lift depression and improve adrenal function.

This highly respected herb is said to develop the 'crown chakra' and synchronize the left and right hemispheres of the brain and therefore used to improve meditation and revitalize the nerves and brain cells.

Gotu Kola is known to strengthen immune function, tonify the adrenals reduce blood pressure and anxiety; 1995 studies showed its effectiveness in destroying cultured tumour cells (in vitro).

Gotu Kola is used in Ayurvedic medicine to cure mental disorders creates balance between the hemispheres of the brain and nourishes the "crown chakra"; it is considered top be one of the major rejuvenative herbs to alleviate disorders associated with old age.

Classified in India as a "Medya Rasayana" (a substance that enhances brain function).

Research: A double blind trial on gotu kola over a 12-week period showed that educable children with severe learning difficulties showed an appreciable improvement in academic performance, an increase in IQ, a marked behavioural improvement and an increased power of concentration and attentiveness. 6.

Active Ingredients: calcium, magnesium, iron, zinc, Vitamins B1, 2,3 and C.

Gotu Kola is a great source of magnesium, vitamin K., calcium and sodium and also contains the saponin glycosides *brahmoside* and *brahminoside* (the herb is often referred to as *Brahmi* - a sanskrit name for The Creator in Indian Mythology - a title it shares with the herb Bacopa – see below). These saponins have diuretic and slightly sedative actions, together with wound healing properties, aiding the stimulation of lipids responsible for healthy skin and hair.

BACOPA: (Bacopa monnieri)

Bacopa is a succulent creeper from the snapdragon family. It has a bitter taste and a warming action. Bacopa acts as a rejuvenative nerve tonic, regenerating mental health, improving memory and promoting intellect. This herb was first recorded in herbal texts around 800 B.C.(*Atharva Veda),* and described in *Susruta Samhita* (one of the earliest Ayurvedic texts) to be effective in treating memory loss, insomnia and decrease the signs of ageing.

TULSI: (Holy Basil, Ocinium sanctum)

In Hindu mythology, Tulsi is the name of a goddess who was re-incarnated as an herb to be offered in worship to Lord Vishnu (*Mahabharata*). The plant is now grown in almost all Hindu homes.

There are three different Tulsi plants used as medicine in India – Rama Tulsi, Krishna Tulsi and Vana (forest) Tulsi – all belong to the same family.

Nutritional Value: - Tulsi is rich in Vitamin A, C, Calcium, Iron, Zinc, Selenium, Manganese and Sodium.

Tridosha: - regulates vata, pitta and kapha (the 3 doshas or body types outlined in Ayurvedic medicine).

Traditional Use: - According to the ancient texts of Ayurveda (*Charak Samhita and Susrut Samhita*) Tulsi is effective in treating coughs and respiratory disorders, poisoning, arthritis and impotence.

Modern Usage: - Tulsi has become increasingly popular as an anti-stress agent with Adaptogenic properties and has compared favourably with herbs such as **Ashwagandha, Panax Ginseng** and **Eleutherococcus** (Siberian Ginseng) [7].

Tulsi has also been shown to have strong anti-oxidant properties and to protect against liver damage caused by free-radical activity [8].

Research has also shown a reduction in fatigue with patients suffering from chronic fatigue syndrome [9].

Acknowledgements: Tulsi – The Mother Medicine of Nature. Dr. Narendra Singh and Dr. Yamuna Hoette – IIHM India 2002.

REJUVENATIVES

Rejuvenation is largely an Eastern concept. It is rarely seen in Western herbalism where there are few tonic herbs (at least in terms of "adaptogens" and "rejuvenatives". The concept of "tonic" in the West is something you take when ill rather than something you use to move from a level of 'wellness' to a level of excellence.

Many of the great tonic herbs were covered on the Chinese Herbal section and earlier in this section (Medhya Rasayan).

I cannot discuss Ayurvedic Medicine without including the following herbs.

ASHWAGANDHA: (Withania somnifera)

An Indian herb used in Ayurvedic medicine and classified as a *rasayana* or elixir. The name Ashwagandha refers to the "vitality of a horse" giving rise to its use as a rejuvenative tonic.

Ashwagandha has a nourishing effect on the nervous and reproductive systems making it useful as both sedative and aphrodisiac (Although this seems like a contradiction. It is found that the majority of cases of sexual dysfunction are aggravated, if not caused, by stress or nervous exhaustion).

A recent double-blind study assessed the effect of Ashwagandha on the ageing process. A group of 101 healthy volunteers, aged between 50 and 59, agreed to take the herb daily for a year. At the end of the year it was found that levels of melanin in hair was increased in the group taking Ashwagandha and calcium loss was significantly lower. 70% of the group using the herb reported increased libido.[10]

Ashwagandha is comparable in Ayurvedic medicine to ginseng in the Chinese pharmacopoeia earning it the name "Indian Ginseng".

AMLA (Emblica officinalis – "Indian Gooseberry")

Amla is a primary rejuvenative tonic that is highly regarded in Ayurvedic Medicine.

Parts Used: Fruit

Energy and Taste: sour, sweetish, cool.

Organs targeted: Heart, Liver, Kidneys.

Active ingredients: Amla contains approximated 20 x more Vitamin C. than oranges in a thermo stable form, making it bio-available and not easily destroyed by drying or heating.

Uses: The sour, fleshy fruit of the Amla tree is classified as being nutritive, digestive, rejuvenative, mild laxative, astringent and disinfectant. Amla is thought to improve resistance, improve the action of the adrenals, assist in the formation of collagen, cartilage, bones and teeth; nourish the blood, improve vision and hair quality. Amla can be used (with other herbs) in cases of liver disease, diabetes, scurvy and anaemia.

Amla is a major ingredient in the Ayurvedic rejuvenative food paste **Chyawan Prash.**

Another compound which includes Amla is the almost legendary **Triphala** ("Three Fruits" Amla, **Haritaki**, **Bibhitaki**) known in India as "The Mother of all Medicines". **Triphala** has a cleansing and harmonising action on the blood, the colon, the liver, the skin and the eyes.

SHATAVARI: (asparagus racemosus, *tian men dong*)

Shatavari (Indian asparagus) has the traditional name "who possesses a hundred husbands" due to its rejuvenative action on the female reproductive organs.
This herb is known to increase fertility and often considered as the female counterpart to **ashwagandha**.

Uses: sexual debility (both sexes), infertility, stomach ulcers, herpes and dysentery.

Notes on Part Two - Ayurveda:

1. Sreejayan.N, Rao MNA Free radical scavenging activity of curcuminoids. Arzneim Forsch Drug Res 1996; 46. 169-71
2. Caseres DD Hancke, JL. Burgos RA. Et al. Use of visual analogue scale measurements (VAS) to assess the effectiveness of standardized Andrographis paniculata extract SHA-10 in reducing the symptoms of common cold. A randomised double blind-placebo study.Phytomedicine 1999; 217-223.
3. www.altcancer.com/andcan.htm
4. Holt, Stephen M.D., Linda Comac, Miracle Herbs Combine with Modern Medicine to Treat Cancer, Heart Disease, AIDS, and More, Caro Publishing Group, 1998.
5. Deng. W.L. Outline of current clinical and pharmacological research on Andrographis paniculata in China. Newsletters of Chinese Herbal Med. 1978;10:27-31
6. Appa Rao et al., 1973
7. Bhargava and Singh 1981
8. Misha et al., 1998.
9. Singh and Abbas, 1995
10. Kuppurajan, k., et al. "Effects of Ashwagandha on the Process of Aging in Human Volunteers". – Journal of Research in Ayurveda 247-258, 1980

PART THREE

THE WESTERN HERBAL TRADITION

THE URBAN HERB GATHERER

Travelling through countries where people still maintain an intimate contact with nature, it is easy to observe local people (generally the womenfolk) gathering healing plants and foods regardless of whether the environment is rural or urban. I well remember seeing groups of women collecting leaves from the tea bushes (**Camellia sinensis**) in the parks of Nanjing, China. These leaves were dried on rooftops and sold to shops in the tea district.

In the U.K. blackberry picking is becoming a forgotten tradition as we move towards a preference for the more exotic (but often less nutritious) fruits offered by our local supermarket.

It is also easy for herbalists, living in the city and classroom trained, to almost forget how herbs grow, or even what they look like in the wild depending on large-scale suppliers of herbs, often rendered into tinctures or powders, before they reach the herbalist.

Yet our local environment can provide us with a great deal of what we need even if that environment is, to a large extent, covered with tarmac and concrete.

As a child born in the last year of the 2nd World War, I remember playing on a bombsite which was taken over by **Buddleia**, **Elder**, **Evening Primrose** and all manner of "herbs" not yet known to me. I marvelled at how nature always finds a way to make even the most devastating scars on the landscape good.

Plant growing seasons often remind us of our needs; **Dandelion** in the spring to help detoxify the liver after a winter of warm and heavy foods. We find elderflower, and yarrow in the summer to cool the blood and open the pores for easier perspiration. Fungi and **rosehips** appear in the autumn to protect the immune system from the coming onslaughts of winter.

In the city we are subject to pollutants from traffic and light industry but we do escape the residues of major crop spraying and massive chemical fertilizing programmes. Our local park or piece of wasteland may not have achieved "organic status" or have the blessing of The Soil Association. But it's all we have on a daily basis. The herbs growing in these places grow naturally, often as "weeds", rather than being cultivated in a way, which may threaten some of their vital properties.

Each year in my local park ("the lung of the city") I gather **hawthorn berries**, rosehips, **lime flowers**, **elderberries** etc. all far from the nearest main road and all free for the taking.

This year my favorite site is a piece of waste ground behind a local pub "beer garden". It is protected from the road by a high fence and a row of large trees.

Nobody visits this place apart from the occasional herb gatherer (only one that I know of) and a few dog owners who tend to keep to the perimeter track. Here I gather **cleavers**, **narrow leaf plantain** (ribwort), the **greater plantain**, **chickweed**, **burdock** and **ground ivy**, the mainstay of my summer salves and teas.

THE HERBS

CLEAVERS: (Galium aparine, clivers, "goose grass")

Cleavers or "Sticky Willy", as we called it as children is in the same order of plants as Sweet Woodruff and Ladies Bedstraw. The plant is best gathered in the spring and early summer. Later in the year it becomes rather stringy and straw-like. When it is young, Cleavers can be pressed in a juicer. The juice is a powerful diuretic and lymphatic cleanser. Although cleavers are not attractive plants and can therefore be classified as "weeds" they have many properties. Apart from their diuretic action cleavers are great blood purifiers (particularly for skin disorders such as psoriasis). They help to soften bladder stones and make a good ointment for scalds, burns and ulceration of the skin.

The astringent nature of cleavers makes it useful in the treatment of excessive menstrual bleeding and diarrhea. It can also be applied as a poultice for sores.

Cleavers seeds are stimulating; they make a good substitute for coffee without the ill effects of caffeine.

So the next time you find this prolific weed wrapped around your favorite garden plants treat it with the respect it deserves.

COREOLUS: (Trametes.versicolor) – 'Turkey Tail Mushroom'

Coreolus is a prolific fungus, which can often be seen covering rotten logs. Although it has a limited fruiting season it survives through most of the year. Its often-vivid bands of colour vary in depth and intensity according to the season or its environment. This fungus is particularly active in the transformation and redistribution of nutrients in the forest.

In China Coreolus is often referred to as "Yun Zhi" or 'Cloud Fungus' and is said to have been a strong influence in the traditional cloud designs on silk garments in oriental cultures. But its most common name is "Turkey Tail" which perfectly describes its appearance.

Coreolus is starting to become quite popular amongst practitioners of Chinese Herbal Medicine due to a flood of research showing this herb to be of benefit in treating serious immune deficiency disorders [1]. including Hepatitis B [2]. and C, AIDS, various cancers and Chronic Fatigue Syndrome (CFS) [3]. In Japan an average of 25% of the annual national expenditure for anti-cancer drugs is devoted to PSK [4]. a coreolus derivative drug that has few or no side effects.

DANDELION: (*Taraxicum officinalis*) White Endive, Lion's Tooth

Dandelion comes from the same plant family as rocket, endive and other bitter salad vegetables. The bitter flavour is most important for the correct function of the gall bladder and other bodily organs yet is almost non-existent in the English diet. Dandelion is very high in nutritive salts such as sodium making it a useful herb in the treatment of blood toxicity, anaemia and skin diseases.

Dandelion was traditionally used for kidney problems (due to its diuretic properties) and for increasing the activity of the liver, spleen and pancreas. The leaves can be added to salads or dried as tea. The root can be added to stir-fries, or roasted and ground as a coffee alternative.

ECHINACEA: (E.purpurea, E.pallida, E.angustifolia, Purple Cone Flower)

Now becoming a household word Echinacea has earned itself a place of prominence in the medicine cabinets of the health conscious as a blood and lymph purifier, an antibiotic, anti-fungal and antiviral remedy.

Echinacea was probably first used by the Pawnee Indians in the treatment of snakebite earning it the name "Kansas Snake Root". It has become popularized as an over the counter medicine due to the work of two pioneering naturopathic herbalists; Dr. Vogel in Europe and Dr. Tierra in the United States.

Echinacea can be used for most mild infections including: sore throats, colds, flu etc. It can be used in syrups for children and it combines well with other herbs such as **Golden Seal**, **Indigo** or **Myrrh**.

Echinacea also contains the major building blocks for the cell protein interferon making it relevant for the treatment of more serious disorders.

This beautiful plant grows easily in the U.K. (providing the slugs give it a chance). Its bright purple flowers are a long lasting addition to herbaceous borders in July and August.

Although it is primarily the roots of the plant, which are, used as medicine the leaves and seeds can be used with some benefit in teas particularly at the onset of viral disorders.

Echinacea is most effective when used in short courses of treatment.

According to American Herbalist Michael Tierra, a leading authority on Echinacea, this herb works through a different pathway from antibiotics inhibiting the enzyme that allows harmful bacteria to penetrate the walls of healthy cells.

Although echinacea is normally promoted as a cold preventative herb, it was traditionally regarded as being most effective in treating infections such as septicemia, venomous bites and gangrene.

I had a personal experience of using massive amounts of echinacea angustifolia tincture externally to treat and cure an infection of the tear duct which had spread to the entire face, causing swelling, blistering and a great deal of pain; hourly applications entirely cleared all infection within five hours.

ELDER: _(sambucus spp., Black Elder, Common Elder, "Pipe Tree")

The elder tree has been used and revered for thousands of years by many healing traditions.

Elder was described by the ancient Greeks as "the tree of medicine" and "the sacred tree".

Elder branches were once used in the manufacture of musical instruments and referred to in the writings of Pliny as "the tree of music".

The flowers have a bitter, cooling energy making them useful in reducing fevers especially in the early stages of colds and flu. Elderflowers are useful in salves for treating burns and skin rashes.

The berries are very high in vitamin C. and contain two compounds that are considered to be effective against several viruses including flu.

An Israeli study showed a 73% success rate in improving flu symptoms with *Sambucol*, a patent syrup rich in elderberries.

Paracelsus described the berries as "plant mercury". As a result modern alchemists use it in reducing the toxins from dental fillings.

As syrup with blueberries I find elderberries a useful base for children's medicines; not only disguising the taste of more bitter herbs but also providing a useful medicinal dimension.

EQUISETUM: (Horsetail)

Horsetail is one of the earliest plants on Earth (Carboniferous Era 300 million years ago). It is an early ancestor of pine trees and one of the plants responsible for coal deposits.

Keyword: Equilibrium

Ruling Planet: Saturn

Represents: Stability, spinal column (simple observation of this plant will show us its potential uses – it appears to be a model for the spine)
Tissues affected: Plasma, blood, fat, bone.
Actions: Diaphoretic, diuretic and haemostatic.
Indications: Oedema, burning of urethra, kidney & gall stones and stomach ulcers.

Promotes the healing of bones, and supplies nutrients (including silica) to bone tissue.

Brightens the eyes and removes blood toxicity.

Acknowledgements:

The Yoga of Herbs – Frawley/Lad – Lotus Press – 1988
Phylak Spagyric Essences – Dr J Naidu – 2007

GARLIC: (Allium sativum)

Known by all herbal traditions as a protecting food/herb and effective in preventing a wide range of pathogens. Garlic aids digestion, improves circulation, lowers blood pressure and has anti-viral, anti-fungal and antiseptic properties.

Recent research (costing more than £20 million) was conducted by a well know cancer charity into the antibiotic properties of certain herbs. The result showed garlic to be an extremely potent antibiotic, antibacterial and antiviral agent. This was known by herbalists for many centuries. Most would have gladly parted with the information for a much more modest fee than that charged by the pharmaceutical scientists.

In Mediterranean countries where garlic is consumed in vast quantities it is shown that there are fewer cases of life threatening disorders including cancers and heart disease.

In ayurvedic medicine it is important to include the six tastes (*rasas*) in the diet; garlic is considered to contain all of the tastes (or flavours) except sour.

Active constituents: sulphur compounds.

History and Folklore: In his writings, the poet philosopher Pliny referred to the ancient Egyptians reverence towards garlic as a deity. The use of garlic in folklore as a protective herb may derive from Homer's Odyssey in which Ulysses used it to escape from being transformed into a pig by Circe.

One of the best ways of using garlic medicinally is with honey. This not only preserves but also modifies the heat of the herb; peeled cloves of garlic (approx 2-3 ounces) are mashed and blended together with half a jar of honey. A teaspoon of the mixture is taken 2-3 times daily to drive out colds, alleviate sore throats and infections of the upper respiratory tract.

GOLDEN SEAL: (Hydrastis Canadensis)

Golden Seal is one of the most powerful, rare and costliest herbs in the western herbal pharmacopoeia. A once prolific member of the Buttercup family (Ranunculacea) Golden Seal is now endangered in the wild and generally quite expensive.

This herb is not easy to grow outside of its native home (the Eastern United States and Canada). It is often substituted with cheaper herbs including **turmeric**, **bloodroot**, **Chinese skullcap** or **coptis**.

Early settlers in the Americas learned of the attributes of Golden Seal from Native American people who used the root in their medicines and the juice as a stain for clothing, skin and weaponry.

Ideally Golden Seal should be treated as an antibiotic and immune stimulant. Therefore it has a restricted usage of 5-7 days each time. Its action is tonic, laxative, cleansing and mildly stimulating; it aids digestion and has a cooling effect on mucous membranes. Golden Seal is a classic liver tonic being rich in berberine, a substance highly prized in Chinese Medicine and found in **gentian**, coptis and other yellow detoxifying herbs.

Contra-indications: Golden seal should be avoided during the early stages of pregnancy.

HAWTHORN: (crataegus spp.)

The medicinal uses of hawthorn were first recorded by Dioscorides (40-80 A.D.).

Its botanical name (crataegus) was derived from the Greek word *kratos*, which means "always having been there".

Although the berries are primarily used all parts of the plant have medicinal and nutritional properties.

Hawthorn has been traditionally used as a heart tonic by peoples as diverse as the American eclectics, the Cherokee nation and the private physician of King Henry IV of France.

Hawthorn berries are used in Chinese medicine where they reduce food stagnation.

The leaves, fresh flowers and buds are shown to exhibit antioxidant activity [5], to have a mild sedative effect [6], and assist in reducing blood pressure [7].

MILK THISTLE - (Silibum Marinarum, Mary Thistle, Marian Thistle, Holy Thistle, Wild Artichoke).

A beautiful plant with dark spiny leaves streaked with milky veins. Milk Thistle can grow to well over a metre high in Southern Europe. The seeds, fruit and leaves are all used for medicinal purposes.

Active Principle: Rich in silymarin (an antioxidant known to be 10 x as powerful as Vitamin E).[8].

Uses: Protects against liver damage including severe poisoning. This latter use has long been recognised in folk medicine with particular regard to its usage to counteract the effects of death cap mushroom *amanita phalloides,* a poison which is fatal in 30% of cases.

Research has shown silymarin to be 100% effective in preventing toxicity from the two peptides present in death cap – which are considered to be the most powerful liver damaging substances known [9].

Other Uses: In cases of viral hepatitis. milk thistle is shown to reverse liver cell damage [10]. To both help prevent and treat gallstones [11].
Milk thistle is shown to reduce leukotriene formation; leukotriene is produced to excess by psoriasis sufferers [12]..

Acknowledgements: The Healing Power of Herbs. Michael .T.Murray N.D. – Prima Health 1992

NETTLE: (Urtica dioica)

A common plant known for its nutritional values

Active ingredients: Nettle is very rich in nutrients such as chlorophyll, beta-carotene, the Vitamins A, C., and E. and Silica. The leaves also contain 5-HTP in appreciable amounts.

Used externally nettle is known to ease rheumatism. Applied to the hair as a rinse it improves colour and cleanses the scalp.

Recent findings suggest that nettle root can be a useful herb in the relief of benign prostatic hyperplasia and aid in the formation of haemoglobin in red blood cells. This common "weed" has a multitude of uses

Uses: Nettle has pain relieving, blood tonifying and diuretic properties. It has been found to treat premature baldness, act as a potent diuretic and tonic herb, aid kidney and bladder function, strengthen blood and expel mucous from the lungs. Nettle also stimulates milk flow making it valuable for cattle farmers.

Nettle assists in the treatment of urticaria, rheumatism and gout; it can also be useful in cases of vaginal yeast infections, anaemia and to dispel melancholia.

Recent research has indicated that nettle may help to alleviate prostate problems in men and increase testosterone availability.

The common stinging nettle is a very adaptable herb. It was certainly a good food source for country people when other vegetables were scarce (and butterflies like it too).

History: Nettles were first introduced to Britain by Caesars troops because they felt it might be necessary to flail themselves with the stinging plant in order to keep warm during the colder winters.

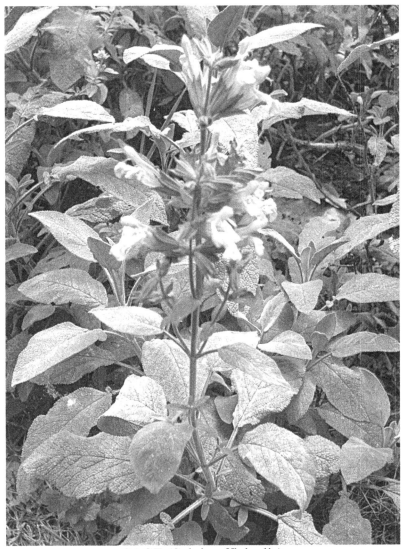

SAGE (Salvia officinalis)

SAGE (Salvia officinalis)

Keywords: Change with decency and sincerity.

Energetic level: Saving remedy.
Sage = Wise. Sage is said to activate intuition and allows us to see the present and not the past.
The word *salvia* comes from the Latin root *salvare, meaning "to heal".*

Physical level:
- Boosts the immune system; it is anti-bacterial, anti-viral and disinfectant.
- Treats respiratory tract infections and digestive disorders.
- Sage is oestrogen like and therefore helps to regulate the menstrual cycle and ease transition through menopause,
- Mild painkiller, eases depression and generally supports the nervous system.
- Helps to fight infections from staphylococcus aereus, E. Coli, candida albicans.
- Sage is specific for calming the heart.

Salvia Divinorum: Used by Mazatec sorcerers to enter other dimensions and access the cause of psychic disturbances and disease.

White Sage: (*salvia apiana)* Is used by Native American peoples to purify their lodges.

Acknowledgements*:*

Dr. J. Naidu. Phylak Sachsen. Switzerland 2005

YARROW: (Achillea millefolium, *gandana* (s), "nosebleed", "Englishman's quinine".

Yarrow (Achillea) was recorded in the Iliad as being used by Achilles to salve the wounds of soldiers in the Trojan wars. Chiron, (the centaur who invented the art of healing) advised Achilles on its use.

Yarrow stalks were well known in ancient Chinese divination (I Ching) in which the laying of the stalks are used to identify the movement of the "Tao" (the way) and help predict destiny.

A powerful herb used throughout the world due to its anti-inflammatory, haemostatic and diaphoretic actions.

Ruler: Venus

Uses: amenorrhea, colds, flu, crohn's disease, high blood pressure, indigestion, ulcers, varicose veins, used topically for nosebleeds, wounds and skin rashes. Yarrow has a slight nervine action and can promote clarity and perception.

Cautions: Yarrow may increase light sensitivity in a small percentage of people. Not to be used (internally) during pregnancy or by lactating mothers.

Notes on Part Three – Western Herbal Tradition:

5. Collins, R.A., Ng, T.B., - Polysaccharpeptide from Coreolus Versicolor has Potential use against Human Immunodeficiency Virus Type 1. Infection. Life Sci. 1997; 60(25) p.383-7.

6. Ying et al. (China) 1987

7. Monro, Dr.Jean. – The Use of Coreolus Versicolor Supplementation in Chronic Fatigue Patients – 3rd International Symposium on Mushroom Nutrition. Milan 2001.

8. Kidd, Dr. Paris. (Ph.D.) – The Use of Mushroom Glucans and Proteoglycans in Cancer Treatment. Alternative Medicine Review. Vol.1. No.1. p.6.

9. Bahorua and others. 1996.

10. Berger. 1984.

11. Lievre and others, 1985.

12. Awang D: Milk Thistle. Can Pharm J 422, 403-404 1995

13. Vogel G, et al: Protection against Amanita phalloides intoxification in beagles. Toxicol Appl Pharm 73 355-362, 1984

14. Benguer J and Carrasco D; Double blind trial of silymarin versus placebo in the treatment of chronic hepatitis. Muench Med Wochenstr.
    119 240 – 260, 1977

15. Nassauto G, et al.: Effect of silibinum on biliary lipid composition. Experimental and clinical study. J. Hepatol

16. Fiebrich F and Koch H: Silymarin an inhibitor of lipoxygenase, Experiment 35, 148-150, 1979

PART FOUR

OTHER HERBAL TRADITIONS:

Interwoven with the larger and more accepted traditions of herbal medicine are the often remote and secretive lineages of Sangomas in Africa, Curenderos in South America, Mexican Sorcerers, the Shamanic cultures of Siberia, Tibet, Western Paganism etc.

Many of these are more occult by nature but also derive from traditions of wholeness, in which the spiritual world is given equal status with the physical.

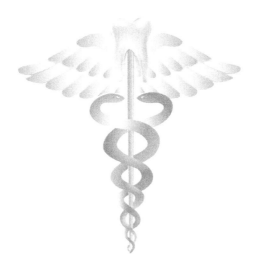

The great medical symbol, The Staff of Hermes used by Hippocrates, was once a winged staff entwined with two serpents or two winged serpents surrounding a staff. The symbol used by the World Health Organization (WHO) and other modern medical institutes now looks more like a mirrored dollar sign than the original ancient symbol. That is only one snake around a plain staff.

Many of the Central American cultures exemplify wholeness in the form of The Plumed Serpent (Quetzalcoatl). Identifying the bird and the snake as the two aspects of Heaven and Earth, or Mystery and Reason. The modern world appears to have lost the mystery replacing it with an "unreasonable amount of reason" in the form of science, technology and materialism.

Parallels can be drawn with the Yin Yang symbol of Chinese philosophy (in which yin or yang cannot exist in isolation but are interdependent) and the Kundalini (*serpent power)* systems of ancient yoga (in which the central *sushumna* channel is intertwined, by the major *Nadis',* the *ida* and *Pingala* as serpents around the central channel.)

The modern medical symbol is almost like the central spine channel entwined by only the *Pingala.* The *Ida* channel can be described as *the mysterious female* and is governed by the moon.

The Western model of medicine is linear, earthbound; we are born, we become sick, we die - end of story.

More traditional approaches are cyclic and evolutionary: we aspire to realisation, to becoming, to oneness. Herbs become a tool in this development. The emphasis is on opening, tonifying and supporting; rather than masking or suppressing.

"Science", is not synonymous with safety, progress or truth (I could spend the rest of this book citing cases to support this point).

NORTH AMERICA:

Although North American herbalism would normally be considered under the heading of Western Herbalism; and many of the great American herbs (including **echinacea**, **golden seal** etc.) have been covered in that section, I feel it necessary to state that the North American culture is distinct in that U.S. practitioners are by nature more pioneering. Many of the herbs used by Native Americans and other "backwoods and mountain people" are unknown or unavailable to European herbalists. Herbs such as **Osha** (ligusticum porterii) and **Chaparral** (creosote bush) are almost without European equivalents.

AMERICAN GINSENG: (Panax quinquifolium)

Panax quinquifolium is another "true" ginseng revered in both east and west. North American Indians originally used it as a remedy for menstrual disorders, fevers and as a "wound herb".

The pioneering backwoodsman, Daniel Boone, managed to gather 15 tons of the roots in 1787 during an expedition up the Ohio River. He first exploited the market for American Ginseng. Since that time a great deal of exploitation has taken place leaving wild American ginseng extremely rare and therefore very expensive.

American ginseng is said to be cooler than its eastern counterpart and has more affinity to the lung nourishing the "Yin" and blood while protecting the "wei qi"*.

It is generally found that American ginseng is richer in ginsenosides than **Asian Panax** and is equally rich in vitamin B., sugars and starches.

* *wei qi* – "protective energy", synonymous with the immune system.

CALIFORNIAN POPPY: (escholzia californica)

The State Flower of California.

Although it is related to the Opium Poppy escholzia contains no opiate alkaloids and is non-addictive.

Actions: analgesic, sedative, nervine.

Uses: insomnia, migraine, depression, anxiety, stress.

No known side effects or drug interactions.

CRAMP BARK: (viburnum opulus, high bush cranberry)

Cramp bark is an age-old remedy. It is used by midwives, herbalists and naturopaths, as a uterine tonic and anti-spasmodic.

Used traditionally by the Iroquois and Ojibwa people for cramping (as its name implies).

Cramp bark was first introduced to the "eclectics" and "shakers" in the mid 19th century.

The First Eclectic dispensary states that cramp bark is very effective in relaxing cramps and spasms and useful in treating asthma, hysteria, pains incident to women during pregnancy etc.[1]

Viburnum opulus is an attractive, ornamental shrub. Its berries provide nutrition for birds and can also be used as a substitute for cranberries.

Acknowledgements:

The American Herbal Pharmacopeia, Roy Upton, Feb. 2000

OREGON GRAPE: (mahonia aquifolium, holly-leaved barberry, mountain grape).

The State Flower of Oregon.

Mahonia is a fast growing, evergreen, prickly leaved shrub. Its sweet smelling yellow flowers give way to the purple, grape-like fruit, which gives it its name.

The berries were traditionally used for poor appetite. The root is used to treat jaundice, arthritis, diarrhoea and to reduce fever.

It is the root that is primarily used medicinally particularly in the treatment of psoriasis [2].

Certain compounds isolated from Oregon grape appear to inhibit the action of lipoxygenase, the enzyme responsible for the over production of skin cells which is the main symptom of psoriasis.

Oregon grape also has a pronounced anti-inflammatory action.

Other uses: chronic candidiasis, parasites, urinary tract infections.

USNEA: Usnea longissima, usnea barbata, hair lichen, *songluo* (Ch.)

It's very hard to place this herb in terms of geographical zone or tradition.

Although it is widely available in The UK and Europe, Usnea is rarely used by herbalists in this part of the world. But it is used a great deal in the United States and known by Eastern and Oriental practitioners.

Usnea was one of the first land plants to emerge and has become one of the widest in application as a powerful medicinal plant.

History: Used for 3,000 years in ancient Egypt, Greece and China to treat unspecified infections 3.

Usnea is something of a natural phenomenon in that it combines the characteristics of both a fungus and algae.

Its Chinese name (*songluo*) refers to *song* - pine (a common host tree) and *luo* - vine or fish net (due to its appearance). In Chinese medicine Usnea is used to treat bronchitis (listed in Oriental Materia Medica as "Phlegm Resolving") and in cancer therapy (particularly for thyroid cancers).

Active Ingredient: usnic acid.

Properties: anti-fungal, antiseptic, antibiotic, antiviral, anti-bacterial, anti-tumour.

Uses: Throat and respiratory tract infections, streptococcal infections, fungal conditions, (including athlete's foot, candida, etc.), urinary tract and vaginal infections, abnormal cervical smear (used in a douche).

External Use: As a dressing for wounds (not only does it assist in controlling bleeding but also helps to prevent infection).

Usnea appears to be much more powerful than penicillin against staphylococcus and streptococcus bacteria. It works by changing cellular metabolism without destroying friendly bacteria or disturbing the natural ecology of the body.

Contraindications: No known contraindications or side effects. (Usnea, like many other herbs, has been used with some success in weight loss programs. This use is due to desperation and often using excessive doses may lead to reactions. This, as with many herb reactions, is due to inappropriate use.)

Acknowledgements:

Hobbs C, Usnea the Herbal Antibiotic, 1990 Botanica Press, Santa Cruz, CA.
Hsu HY, et al., Oriental Materia Medica: A Concise Guide, 1986 Long Beach CA.
Smith J, The Power of Parasitic Plants: URHP newsletter 2005

CENTRAL & SOUTH AMERICA:

These cultures are well known for great herbs of power, from the psychotropics of the shamanic tradition to the commonly used stimulants (coffee, guarana, cola vera, chilli, cocaine etc.) and some more "user friendly" herbs. The Amazon rain forest holds a wealth of botanical treasures much of which is still undiscovered

CAT'S CLAW: - (Uncaria tomentosa - *Una de gato*)
A high climbing vine found in the highlands of the Peruvian Amazon where it is traditionally used by Anashaninka Indians. They know it as "The opener of the way".

It is known as Cat's Claw due to its claw-like thorns, which resemble the claws of a cat.

Properties: ant-viral, anti-oxidant, metabolic tonifier.

Parts used: Inner bark

Uses: To aid the bodies defence system, support intestinal health, to help treat gastritis, ulcer, haemorrhoids, crohn's disease, IBS etc. Cat's Claw can also be used in cases of depression, M.E., cancer, PMS, stress, asthma and all forms of herpes.

Active ingredients: Include "quinovic acid glycosides" (which appear to have high "free radical" scavenging properties) and *isopteridin* (a powerful immune stimulant).

GRAVIOLA: (anona muricata, *guanabana*)

Graviola is a small evergreen tree. The bark, fruit, leaves and the indigenous population of the Amazon rain forest for centuries to treat heart disease, lung and liver problems and arthritis has used roots.

In the 1970s a well known pharmaceutical company, together with the National Cancer Institute, poured large amounts of money and resources into years of research into Graviola as an anti cancer drug.

Research indicated that graviola had great potential in treating lung, breast, prostate, liver and stomach cancers.

It was found in laboratory tests that two chemicals in Graviola selectively killed colon cancer cells. It is 10,000 times more effectively than *adriamycin*, a commonly used chemotherapy drug [4].

After seven years of trying to isolate and duplicate these two chemicals, the pharmaceutical company found replication to be impossible. They couldn't sell the original extracts profitably due to patent licensing laws.

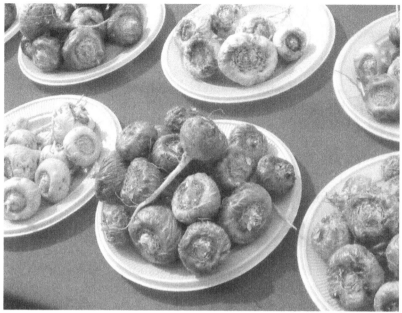

Various roots of organic maca

MACA: (Lipidium Peruvianum)

From the mountains of the Andes and closely related to the radish than to any other plant. It contains no fewer than 55 beneficial phyto-chemicals including a wide range of vitamins, minerals, amino acids and other useful nutrients 5.

Maca has been used traditionally since the time of the Incas (3000 years) and is still commonly traded as an energy tonic throughout Peru.

This rare "radish" is known to build muscle, elevate mood and regulate hormones. No wonder it is gaining recognition as a healthy alternative to coffee and earning itself the pseudonym "Peruvian Ginseng".

PAU D'|ARCO; (lapacho impetiginosa, *taheeba,* trumpet tree, *tabebuia,* "divine bark".

Pau D'Arco is a tropical tree which grows throughout Central and South America and is also found in the Caribbean.

The tree can grow to around 30 metres tall. It is immune to attack from the fungi so common in rain forest areas; making it an obvious herb to use as protection from fungal and yeast infections.

Pau D'Arco has been used medicinally since the time of the ancient Inca and Aztec tribes.

Part Used: Inner bark.

Active ingredients: Lapachol (anti-tumour), napthoquinones (known to stop multiplication of the malaria parasite), Quercetin and other flavinoids.

Uses: Effective against bacteria, fungal, viral, parasite and yeast infections. Pau D'Arco is included in popular modern treatments for candidiasis.

Used for centuries as a treatment for cancer, lupus and other disorders.

Safety: Although Pau D'Arco has been used for decades in South America as a cancer cure; large doses of the herb (on its own) can be mildly toxic. Ideally Pau D'Arco (in high doses) should be combined or alternated with other herbs. As with many herbs, the herb itself is recommended; the use of isolated lapacho compounds, may be inappropriate.

Acknowledgements;
Medicinal Herbs of the Rain Forest. Rita Elkin M.H. Woodland Publishing 1997

Prescriptions for Herbal Healing. Phyllis Balch. Avery 2002

QUEBRA PEDRA: (Phyllanthrus spp., Chanca Pedra, Rock Bush, Stone breaker, Bhumiamlaki, Yerba de la Nina, Yerba de Quinina, Zhen Zu Cao).

Although I was familiar with this herb in my work with Ayurvedic medicine it was not until much later in Madeira that I first found it in the store of a market herb trader and became aware of its potential.

Quebra Pedra (Portuguese for stone breaker) appears to crop up in all traditions with similar climatic zones from: The Caribbean to The Azores, From Nepal to Peru, from China to Cuba.

This herb is a valuable addition to any kidney or liver cleanse combinations,

Traditional Usage: To expel stones, support kidney function, hepato-protective, and digestive, to lower cholesterol, blood pressure, and blood sugar, mildly laxative, to expel worms and kill unfriendly bacteria.

Contra-Indications: Like many cleansing herbs Quebra Pedra should be avoided during pregnancy.

SUMA: (Pfaffia paniculata)

A large climbing vine, from the amaranth species found throughout South America particularly in the region of the Amazon basin. Suma has been used for centuries by indigenous tribes but was not recorded by botanists until 1826 when they were introduced to the herb by its Spanish name *para toda* ("for all things"). This powerful herb has been found to improve all kinds of conditions and has no known toxicity.

Rich in the plant hormones sitosterol, and stigmasterol (which are said to encourage oestrogen production). Suma has become popular as a hormone regulator.

The saponins in suma root (including pfaffosides, pfaffic acids and glycosides 6.) have been clinically demonstrated to inhibit tumour cell melanomas. This gives rise to two patented anti-tumour medicines in Japan. U.S. patents targeting skin, hair and even sickle cell anaemia have been filed using suma derivatives.

THE SOUTH PACIFIC:

I cannot exclude this remote island culture and one of its key herbs used ceremonially for centuries.

Growing up in The UK I became a little disillusioned with Western Herbalism, although it was obviously a profound and ancient system of healing. I was aware of the restrictions placed on it over the centuries by religious, governmental and pharmaceutical interests. I inherited the caution this led to in practitioners of the art.

I observed a great Ayurvedic Doctor at work in Western Fiji and realized that this was a much less restricted tradition (and one which I was later to study in greater depth). But it was the work of a local Fijian "Witch Doctor" that inspired me to eventually train as a herbalist.

He lived in a remote jungle village where he shared his grass hut with a tame flying fox. It hung like a battered umbrella from the bamboo lintel above the doorway and glanced sleepily at visitors.

Always, as with all traditional Fijians, we were greeted with a coconut shell bowl, or two, filled with **Yagona.** This had an immediate relaxing effect, leaving the mind alert, the tongue mildly numb and the rest of the body decidedly "chilled" - an ideal way to observe a master at work without questions or judgement.

KAVA-KAVA: (Piper methysticum, yaqona)

Used in Fiji and other Pacific cultures as a ceremonial herb to bestow welcome and respect. It is normally prepared as a drink. Both roots and twigs are pounded into a mash in water and strained through a cloth (traditionally made from the fibres of wild hibiscus).

Actions: Kava-Kava has a relaxing effect which is analgesic, anti-convulsive and sleep prolonging (especially if sleep is normally disturbed by pain, or muscular stiffness).

Kava-kava also has anti-fungal properties.

I find it interesting to note that before it was banned in Europe, sales of Kava-Kava were exceeding those of the popular sedative Prozac (a pharmaceutical drug currently under investigation).

Averse side effects from Kava-Kava tend to occur when taking extremely high doses of standardised extracts of the herb over long periods of time. Subjects with heavy alcohol, tobacco and pharmaceutical drug usage generally reported the negative effects of Kava-Kava use. This makes it difficult to assess what is responsible. 7.

Acknowledgements:

The Healing Power of Herbs. Michael T Murray N.D. Prima Health. U.S.A. 1995

HAWAIIAN NONI: (morinda citrifolia, "Indian mulberry", kura)

Although the fruit is the most used part of this tall evergreen Polynesian bush; every part of the plant has medicinal properties. The leaves are analgesic, the roots lower blood pressure and the flowers are anti-inflammatory.

The bitter, rancid smelling, fruits, possess all the above properties, together with being anti-bacterial, antibiotic, laxative, sedative and tonic.

Traditionally, the fruits are picked before they ripen, then left in the sun to soften, mashed and strained through cloth.

Noni, in various forms, has become a well-respected tonic throughout the west.

The biochemist, Dr. Heinicke, a foremost researcher into the benefits of noni has isolated a key ingredient which activates the alkaloid Xeronine.

Xeronine in turn activates the enzymes responsible for health maintenance.

A great deal of research has indicated the place of noni in the fight against several disorders including lung cancer. 8.

Acknowledgements:

Hawaiian Noni. Rita Elkins, M.H. – The Woodland Health Series. 1998.

THE MIDDLE EAST:

UNANI TIBB, AVICENNA &
FRAGRANCES OF THE SOUL

According to the Unani Tibb system, as with all traditional medicine systems, sickness is described as a state of imbalance. A part of the journey to wholeness; true health or well-being only occurs when the body is in a state of total harmony. Health (wholeness) is a state in which the four Humours (with blood, phlegm, yellow bile, & black bile) are in a state of relative balance. (I say "relative" because one, or more humours will naturally dominate according to a person's body type as with the *doshas* in Ayurvedic medicine).

Apart from the four Humours, a Unani Tibb practitioner will also assess The four Primary Intemperaments, i.e.: excess of heat, excess of cold, excess of moisture, excess of dryness; and prescribe foods, herbs and oils to return the system to a state of balance.

The founder of Unani Tibb was Hakim Abu Ali Abdullah Hussein Ibn Sina known in the west as Avicenna.

Avicenna was born in 980A.D, near the city of Bokhara (then part of Afghanistan); he was not only influenced by the work of Hippocrates but learned a great deal from the healing traditions of India, China and The Middle East.

By the age of 14, Avicenna was appointed the chief physician of the royal court and later wrote 276 major works covering virtually every subject area. His unparalleled fame came largely from the five volumes entitled The Canon of Medicine The Encyclopaedia Britannica regards this as, "The most famous book in the history of medicine in both east and west".

The Canon of Medicine lists 282 plants used as medicines. The list includes herbs from The Middle East, Europe, China, India and Tibet.

KHALONJI: (Nigella sativa, Nigella damascena, black cumin seed, "love in the mist", *habbat al barakah*)

" The cure for every disease except death"-
Mohammed Origins: **Syria**

Although kalonji is of Middle Eastern origin it will grow very easily in many parts of the world. Once established it is difficult to get rid of. But its cloud of blue flowers is a pleasant sight in any spring garden.

Qualities: Hot & Dry (2nd Degree)

Properties: Abortifacient, emmenagogue, diuretic, carminative, stimulant.

Traditional Use: for bronchial complaints, paralysis, piles, eruptive skin conditions, intestinal disorders, kidney and liver function, immune support.
   A decoction of the seeds is used to promote contractions of uterus after birth and encourage breast milk.

Avicenna was the first person to perfect the art of distillation of plant essences

He found that these essences, or *Attars*, were very effective in treating emotional, and spiritual disorders as the soul of the plant is able to enhance the soul (*Ruh)* of the patient via the heart.
   Avicenna considered all Attars to be cardiac tonics. He included 40 attars in his list of 63 cardiac drugs.
   He saw the heart to be the seat of the production of vital force and a direct link to pure spirit. This is not dissimilar to the concept of *shen* in Chinese medicine.

The word *Attar* is an Arabic word meaning fragrance or essence.

The difference between eastern attars and western aromatherapy oils is that the attar is produced for its particular fragrance using the finest plant materials without alcohol or any type of solvent. It was felt that alcohol would destroy the vital force of the plant.

Enflourage is the most common extraction process. In this procedure plant materials are pressed between sheets of glass or rolled in stone troughs to extract their essence.

The most popular botanical substances used in Attar preparation, include: Oud, Rose, Saffron, Jasmine, Amber, Sandalwood, Myrrh, Tuberose and Frankincense.

OUD: (Oudh, eaglewood, agarwood, aquillaria species, jin-koh, Ch'en Xiang, "wood of God")

A resinous wood taken from ancient trees. The resin is produced as a natural immune response to parasitic growths and therefore mainly found in infected trees; as a result Oud is exceedingly rare, and expensive.

Oud is highly cherished and traded amongst Unani, Ayurvedic and Chinese healers, exotic oil traders, alchemists and religious leaders.

Oud is referred to in Biblical and other religious texts. It is known by the name *Aloes* in The Old Testament and *ahalim* in the Hebrew texts.

The resinous wood is burned on charcoal; it releases a perfume that inspires a relaxed positivity. Oudh can also be purchased as attar.

Oud attar is often priced in the region of £50 - £5000 per dram depending on age, quality and origin.

Much of the Oud available is either falsified using other botanicals or illegally poached from conservation areas. Some Oud is cultivated although this rarely has the "depth" of that coming from older trees.

The perfume of Oud attars vary from a rich almost fecal smell, to sweeter spicier, fragrances.

Medicinal Uses: Stimulant, tonic, calmative, eases pain, useful for lung disorders (including asthma, TB etc), calms the heart, nourishes spirit.

> *"A disciple asked a Sufi Shaykh how to deal with emotional disturbances.He was told to wear high quality Oud attar at 4pm each day, sit in a quietcorner and reflect on the immeasurable generosity, kindness and mercy ofthe One who created this fragrance."*

Acknowledgements:

Qasi Shaikh Abbas Borhany Yemen Times, Issue 863,Volume 13

The Rose : *'The Queen of the Garden of Paradise'*

The Rose was first cultivated for its medicinal and ceremonial use in ancient Persia. From there it spread across Mesopotamia to Palestine, Asia Minor and on to Greece and Western Europe.

The name "rose" was derived from the Roman word for red (*rodon*). It was the name given to the Damascene red rose which was thought to have sprung from the blood of Adonis.

Sappho (600 B.C.) heralded the rose as: *"the Queen of Flowers"*.

The rose is known as *"the flower of secrets"*. The Roman term *"sub rosa"* relates to confidential meetings held under a rose emblem. The plaster ceiling centerpiece still being referred to as *"a rose"*.

Rosa Rugosa, a very old rose species has five petals, in pentagonal symmetry. It is said to relate to the five pointed star Venus, used as a guide by navigators and synonymous with womanhood and the Goddess.

More than a hundred species of roses are used in medicine for their tonic, astringent and carminative properties. It is used in gargles, enemas, teas and salves to treat everything from mouth ulcers to uterine bleeding, etc.

Roses are rich in the bioflavinoid Quercetin, Vitamin C and many other nutrients.

It is said that mediaeval alchemists, including Nostradamus, used extracts of rose to treat and contain The Black Death. The nursery rhyme *"Ring a ring of roses"* dates back to that time.

Attar of Roses, known by Avicenna to be cold and dry in the 2nd degree is commonly used in all cases where heat is the major problem.

- Combined with sweet almond oil for ulcers in the mouth or throat.
- Massaged between the shoulder blades for difficulty swallowing.

- Applied to the gums for grinding of the teeth.
- Mixed with garlic oil and vinegar for toothache.
- Rose water for bad breath, sties and inflammation of the eyes.
- Rose Oil rubbed into the nasal passages, for sneezing and itching of the nose.

Acknowledgements:

Much of the background material for this section was drawn with gratitude from works by Hakim G.M.Chishti: including: - The Traditional Healer. Thorsons Publishing Group. 1988. and Medicines for the Soul: Spiritual Aromatherapy Practitioner's Handbook by Hakim G.M. Chishti, N.D. (permission granted).
Brief history of the rose drawn from: A Modern Herbal. Mrs M Grieve. Penguin Books. 1980
The Da Vinci Code. Dan Brown. Corgi Books. 2004 - for fictional but thought provoking input.

Notes on Part Four – Other Traditions:

1. Tilford G L Edible and Medicinal Plants of the West Missoula, M T: Mountain Press Publishing Co. 1997 148-9
2. Weisenauer M, Ludtke R,.Mahonia aquifolium in patients with psoriasis vulgaris.
3. King and Newton, 1852
4. Kimura Y, et al (Japan) 1983 and Arch S, (Japan) 1986
5. I Garro, 1972 and Denni A., et al, 1994
6. Nishimoto N, Shiobara Y, Inoue S, et al. Three ecdysteroid glycosides from Pfaffia resinoids, Phytochem. 1988: 27:1665-8.
7. Matthews J D, et al, Effects of heavy usage of Kava-Kava on physical health. 1988.
8. A. Hirazumi, E. Furusawa, S.C.Chou, and Y. Hokama, "Anti cancer activity of Morinda Citrifolia on intra periotneally implanted Lower lung carcinoma in syngenic mice." PROC. WEST. PHARMACOL (37): 1994, 145-148.

CONCLUSION

In this book I have attempted to outline some of the salient points that relate to a selection of herbs from various cultures.

Some of these herbs are endangered due to environmental factors, over harvesting and other considerations. Others may be restricted, although I avoided mentioning the majority of these, and others may be threatened by legislation.

Current EU legislation seems to be aimed at making a great majority of herbal and nutritional supplements unavailable as "over the counter" (OTC) medicines and restricting their availability to both practitioners and the general public.

The MHRA (Medicines and Healthcare Regulatory Authority) considers that any herb without 15-30 years recorded use in the European Union should not be available. This in spite of the fact that non-European cultures have used herbs as safe medicines for centuries before the concept of Europe existed.

Dangers do exist regarding excessive dosages, combining certain herbs with pharmaceutical drugs and incorrect identification of certain plants. Probably the worst-case scenario of wrongful identification in recent years was with a member of the **aristolachia** species (a large plant family). This led to serious side effects, resulting in all aristolachia species plants being banned in herbal formulae (a wise precaution under the circumstances).

Most herb suppliers that I have been in touch with over the years are thorough, knowledgeable and have integrity. However, there are charlatans in all professions and individuals who are willing to make money from the suffering of others.

The best of the OTC ("over the counter") supplement companies are advised by qualified herbalists and/or nutritionists. But some simply "Jump on a band wagon" and sell low quality, low dosage products or inappropriate, ill-considered complexes based on what is popular rather than what is safe and/or effective. Unfortunately many people turn to the media rather than to a health care professional for advice on health.

With regard to combinations; there are standard tried and tested formulae used by practitioners of traditional herbal medicine. These can be modified to fit an almost endless array of symptoms and individuals.

(Practitioners of traditional herbal medicine usually focus more on "treating the person, rather than the disease").

As herbal formulae are based largely upon the "energetic" properties of the herbs there is no reason why herbs from many different herbal cultures cannot be combined in one formula.

Perhaps *"Planetary Herbology"*, (as coined by master herbalist, Michael Tierra), is a useful idea in that it upholds the concepts of wholeness, essential in healing and breaks down a great deal of the "separatism" that leads to so many problems in the world.

For many years the western herbal pharmacopoeia has included such eastern herbs as **Panax** and **Eleutherococcus.** Chinese materia medica includes **dandelion, hawthorn, rosehip** etc. Ayurvedic herbs are littered with spices which the average western household has in its food cupboard; and in turn many of our English garden plants were brought from the Himalayas.

Unani Tibb, Middle Eastern medicine, drew from both the classical western materia medica of Hippocrates and the herbs and knowledge brought through Persia, Syria and Mesopotamia by traveling traders from Asia and The Orient.

There are differences in the philosophies underlying different approaches to healing but there is a strong thread that unites them all.

It is often sensible to use herbs from different traditions in one formula, as there are certain qualities where different herbal traditions excel:

- India – a yogic meditative culture whose health systems are centered on "Digestive Fire." India has some of the best "herbs for the mind" and some of the best carminatives.
- China – a culture from which we have a range of martial arts. China has some of the best tonic and adaptogenic herbs such as: **Ginseng, Astragalus, Schizandra, etc.**
- The western tradition of herbalism has some of the best laxatives and diuretics – (I don't know what this says about the west. Do we still have the belief that we are "sinners needing to be purged"?)

It is often the case that a balanced herbal formula will require tonic, carminative, sedative and diuretic herbs; so why not combine the best from each culture?

Western herbal medicine has little to compete with **Chinese ginseng** or **Indian holy basil**. The Eastern traditions could benefit greatly from some of the western "wayside weeds".

The West has benefited a great deal from eastern philosophies and physical practices. The East has benefited from western science and technology. All traditions have something to offer to the whole of humankind.

The blending of eastern and western values is exemplified in the Chinese yin yang symbol, the plumed serpent of Mexican shamanism or even the right and left hemispheres of the brain.

It is my hope that this small book will help to unite traditions of healing and lead to a better understanding of the power of herbs.

GLOSSARY OF TERMS
(Terms not covered by this list should be found in the body of the text.)

Abortifacient – Abortion inducing.

Adaptogen – An herb that enables the body to achieve homeostasis.

Analgesic – Relieves pain.

Antipyretic – Reduces body temperature.

Antispasmodic - Calms muscle spasm.

Apaureshaya - Coming from a Divine source.

Atharva Veda - A Vedic text dealing with incantation (circa 200 A.D).

Attar - Perfume, essence.

Bioflavonoid – A nutrient, which protects cell and capillary walls.

Carminative – Decreases stomach spasm and flatulence.

Charak Samhita – Early Ayurvedic text circa 600 B.C.

Chyawan Prash – A restorative tonic created by Rishi Chyawan.

Crown Chakra – Energy vortex relating to the pineal.

Diaphoretic – Promotes sweating.

Diuretic – Increase urination.

Doshas – Body types based on combination of elements: **Pitta** = fire +water, **Vata** = air + ether, **Kapha** = earth and water.

Emmenagogue – Promote menses.

Expectorant – Expels mucous.

Haemostatic – Stabilizes blood.

Ida – A Major "Nadi" or energy pathway to the left of the spinal column

Jing – Relates to "Kidney Essence".

Mantra – Sacred sound

Medya Rasayana – A substance that enhances brain function.

Mudras – lit. "Seal" – ritual hand gestures.

Pingala – A major "nadi" (energy pathway) to right of spinal column.

Polysaccharide – A carbohydrate made up of linked sugar molecules.

Qi – Relates to flow of energy

Quetzalcoatl – Aztec sky god.

Rasas – Tastes or flavours.

Rasayana – A restorative elixir.

Rig Veda – Earliest Vedic text (hymns).

Ruh – Soul or spirit (Arabic)

Sankhya – lit. "Pertaining to number". An Indian philosophical system.

Shen – Spirit relates to the heart (Chinese)

Spleen – In Chinese medicine the term "spleen" refers to a major energetic function and is not to be confused with the western idea of the spleen as a relatively insignificant organ.

Sushumna – A major "nadi" (energy channel) running through the spine.

Susrut Samhita – Early Ayurvedic text circa 800 B.C.

Upangas – lit. "Upper, limbs" relating to the six systems of Indian philosophy.

Yin & Yang – The polarities in Chinese philosophy.

INDEX OF HERBS

BIBLIOGRAPHY
**(Smaller publications referred to but not listed
below are acknowledged in the body of the text or
in the chapter notes.)**

Balch, Phyllis. Prescriptions for Herbal Healing, Avery, 2002.
Bleument / Lui. Jiaogulan: China's Immortality Herb, Torchlight Publishing, 1999.
Castaneda, Carlos. The Second Ring of Power, Pocket Books
Chishti, G.M. The Traditional Healer, Thorson's, 1988.
Chishti, G.M. Eastern Spiritual Aromatherapy – Course Handbook, 2002 (unpublished)
Duke, James. A. The Green Pharmacy, Rodale Press, Pennsylvania, 1997
Elkin, Rita. Hawaiian Noni, Woodland Publications, 1988
Elkin, Rita. Medicinal Herbs of the Rain Forest, Woodland Publications, 1987.
Frawley/Lad. The Yoga of Herbs, Lotus Press 1988
Grieve, M. A Modern Herbal, Penguin Books, 1980
Hobbs, Christopher. Medicinal Mushrooms, Botanica Press. 1986
Hobbs, C. Usnea the Herbal Antibiotic, Botanica Press, 1990.
Murray, Michael. The Healing Power of Herbs, Prima Health, 1992
Naidu, J. Phylak Spagyric Essences, (unpublished, ongoing) 2007
Singh/Hoette. Tulsi- The Mother Medicine of India, IIHM, India, 2002.
Smith/Tierra. Earth Force Training Manual re Planetary Formulas, (unpublished, ongoing).
Stamets, Paul. Mycomedicinals, MycoMedia, 2002.
Teaguarden, Ron. Radiant Health – The Ancient Wisdom of Chinese Tonic Herbs, Warner Books, 1988
Tierra, Michael. The Way of Chinese Herbs, Pocket Books, 1998.
Tierra, M. The Way of Herbs, Pocket Books, U.S.A. 1998.
Tilford, G.L. Edible and Medicinal Plants of West Missoula, Mountain Press, 1997.
Upton, Roy. The American Herbal Pharmacopoeia, 1999.
(ongoing work, with many published monographs).

Lightning Source UK Ltd
Milton Keynes UK
UKOW06f0147020316

269454UK00017B/628/P